By the same author
in
Orient Paperbacks
Yoga in Daily Life (Illus)

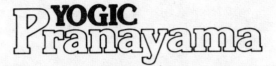

YOGIC Pranayama

Breathing for long life & good health

K.S. Joshi, *M. Sc., M.A., Ph. D.*
Head of the Dept. of Yoga,
University of Sagar, M.P.

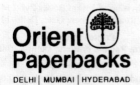

Orient Paperbacks

DELHI | MUMBAI | HYDERABAD

www.orientpaperbacks.com

ISBN 81-222-0089-3

1st Published 1982
12th Printing 2004

Yogic Pranayama:
Breathing for Long Life and Good Health

Cover design by Gurunathan for Vision Studio

Published by
Orient Paperbacks
(A division of Vision Books Pvt. Ltd.)
Madarsa Road, Kashmere Gate, Delhi-110 006

Printed in India at
Rashtra Rachna Printers, Delhi-110 092

Cover Printed at
Ravindra Printing Press, Delhi-110 006

Contents

Cure of disorders 138

Appendix:
A Keep Fit-Yoga Routine 178

Illustrations

1

What is Pranayama ?

Pranayama is an important, yet little known part of Yoga. Its techniques have been practised for centuries by ardent students of Yoga in remote ashrams, and have been preserved for us through many generations both in practice and in handwritten books. Until recently, this art and science of Yogic breathing was almost completely unknown to the common man like many other ancient Indian arts. Those who knew it used to be very reluctant to share their knowledge and experience with anyone, unless a student proved by tests that he was ready to receive it. During the last three decades, however, this situation has changed, and subjects such as Yoga, pranayama, meditation, and even Kundalini, are being discussed all over the world, not only by Yoga teachers, but also by the general public and by scientists. More recently, various techniques of Yoga have begun to attract the attention of physicians, therapists, and medical consultants. It is common to find both patients and doctors who can narrate their own experiences about the cure of various diseases by using Yoga techniques. It has been proved beyond doubt that pranayama is a very important means for preventing and curing many ailments. It is this factor more than any other that has prompted the writing of this book. Its aim is to bring the traditional knowledge of this great art of the common man, so that it can be used without much external help for the maintenance as well as the restoration of health. It is hoped that by reading this book the reader will be well equipped to keep diseases away by using the age-old techniques of pranayama.

Pranayama is the fourth part of the eight-fold Yoga described in the *Yogasutra* of Patanjali. This is the most authoritative book on yoga. It was written, or according to many experts on the subject, in the second century before Christ. The eight limbs of yoga mentioned in Patanjali's system are: (1) Yama, (2) Niyama, (3) Asana, (4) Pranayama, (5) Pratyahara, (6) Dharana, (7) Dhyana, and (8) Samadhi.

Pranayama is also mentioned in the Gita, which is, by far, the most popular book on yoga. But a detailed account of how pranayama is to be practised is not found in the Gita or the *Yogasutra*. For that we have to turn to the texts of Hathayoga and to some later Upanishads which are called Yoga-upanishads. These texts are of approximately the fifteenth century A.D., and later. It should not be concluded from this that the techniques of pranayama have been known only for the last five hundred years. Many direct and indirect references to pranayama, what it can do, why it is practised, and what its importance is, occur in Vedic literature, in ancient Upanishads, Smritis, Puranas, and treatises such as the *Yogavasistha*. This shows that a knowledge of pranayama and its practices was known since the time of the Vedic rishis. But it seems quite certain that the practice of pranayama was taught to very few. It was never widespread. Even the few who learned it, followed it more as a part of religious observances than as a discipline for the body and mind.

The credit for making the practice of pranayama popular as a discipline in its own right and as a means for maintaining the health of the body and mind goes to the followers of Hathayoga. They gave it a place of great importance among the practices of Hathayoga, and it was they who described various techniques of pranayama, emphasizing the utility of each of them. Hathayoga is said to consist of four main types of practices, namely, asana, pranayama, mudras, and nadanusandhana, that is, being aware of the inner sounds. These four types of practices are supposed to lead ultimately to the state of samadhi, which would bestow upon the individual aspirant of yoga absolute knowledge, or self-knowledge, which in its turn leads to emancipation or liberation from the cycle of rebirths.

When we start thinking about pranayama with this background some questions arise in our mind. We shall discuss them here one by one. The questions are as follows:

1. What is pranayama?
2. How did pranayama originate?
3. Why do we breathe at all?

4. Why should we control the breath?

5. What can pranayama do?

In a way, this whole book is an attempt to provide answers to these questions. But here we shall consider them from the point of view of a beginner, in order to form a general idea about pranayama, so that details mentioned in the subsequent chapters could be understood more clearly.

Pranayama is control of breath

In simple terms pranayama may be called the control of the breath. Its essence lies in the modification of our normal process of breathing. Breathing is an act in which we take air from the atmosphere into our lungs, absorb the oxygen from it into our blood, and expel the air again into the atmosphere together with carbon-di-oxide and water vapour. This act of inhalation and exhalation is repeated every four to five seconds. Thus normally we breathe about fifteen times every minute, each time taking about 500 ml. of air into the lungs. So we inhale and exhale approximately seven litres of air per minute. Every modification of this normal breathing process would not count as pranayama. The normal breathing pattern shows marked changes under various conditions. For instance, while we are lifting or carrying loads, walking uphill, running, or doing any physical exercise we breathe more rapidly and more forcefully. At high altitudes, in a rarefied atmosphere our breathing becomes heavy. Its pattern changes with emotional excitement and in the case of disorders such as asthma, tuberculosis, bronchitis and other lung affections. Modification of breathing under these conditions is brought about involuntarily, and perhaps without awareness of it unless there is difficulty in breathing. In fact we are hardly ever aware of the fact that we are breathing.

Pranayama consists of modifications of the breathing process which we bring about deliberately and consciously. We can modify breathing in three different ways:

1. By inhaling and exhaling rapidly, taking shallow breaths.
2. By inhaling and exhaling slowly, taking long or deep breaths.
3. By stopping the act of breathing altogether.

The first way of modifying breathing is not usually included in pranayama proper, although it is sometimes closely associated with it. The second and third ways mentioned above do belong to the domain of pranayama. In fact, pranayama practice may very well be summarised in these two ways.

There is one more condition to be fulfilled if any breathing modification is to be called pranayama. That is regarding the posture. Pranayama is practised in a sitting posture. There are about half a dozen postures available for this purpose. They are called meditational postures, because they are very suitable for meditation. The most renowned among them is Siddhasana. The simplest and most comfortable and less strenuous is Swastikasana. Padmasana is the one which is most recommended traditionally for pranayama. We shall describe these postures in detail in a later chapter. It may be enough to mention here that pranayama is defined by Patanjali as a modification of breathing in a sitting posture which is steady and comfortable. Such a posture is an essential part of pranayama.

Thus pranayama is a complex act in which after assuming a suitable posture the student inhales and exhales slowly, deeply, and completely, and also stops the breath. Inhalation in pranayama is called *puraka*, which literally means 'the act of filling', Exhalation is called *rechaka*, meaning 'the act of emptying'. Retention of breath is called *kumbhaka. Kumbha* means a water pot. Just as a water pot holds water when it is filled with it, so in kumbhaka the breath is held after filling the lungs. Actually, kumbhaka can be practised in two ways. We can hold the breath in after a puraka, or we can hold the breath out after a rechaka. The first variety is recommended much more in traditional books. It is called *abhyantara kumbhaka* or *antah-kumbhaka*. The second variety of kumbhaka is called *bahya-kumbhaka*.

In traditional writings the two words pranayama and kumbhaka are often used as synonymous words. This may be explained by the fact that kumbhaka is the most important part of pranayama. There seems to be a difference of opinion among experts about whether a modified way of breathing which does not include any kumbhaka can be called pranayama at all. For instance, if one practises only puraka and rechaka without any kumbhaka, then can it be said that one is practising pranayama?

Some writers, who have argued that kumbhaka is an indispensable part of pranayama, would insist that mere puraka and
rechaka do not form pranayama. But there are others who do
not agree with this way of defining pranavama.

How did pranayama originate

Howsoever we define pranayama, that is to say, whether we
make kumbhaka an indispensable part of it or not, one essential
feature of pranayama according to any definition, is, that it
involves a control of breath. Breath is called *prana* in Sanskrit.
Prana also means the soul. In the word pranayama prana does
not mean the soul, but the breath. The association of these two
meanings of the word prana is obviously quite close. Breath
and life go together. When any living being dies, breathing stops.
This close association between breath and the soul attracted the
attention of the ancient Aryans more, because they believed in
a cycle of rebirths, until the soul became emancipated by attaining *moksha* or *mukti*.

This is called the belief in transmigration of the soul. This
belief is very clearly expressed in the following *slokas* of the
Bhagavadgita:

"Just as one throws away old clothes and takes new ones,
so, too, the soul, i.e., the dweller in the body, leaves old bodies
and enters into new ones." (Gita: II.29)

"Whosoever is born is sure to die, and one who dies is sure
to be born again. This cycle is unavoidable. Hence it is no use
being unhappy about it." (Gita: II.27)

The observation that so long as one is breathing one is living, and that when the breath stops life comes to an end,
accompanied by the belief that the soul transmigrates from birth
to birth, must have played an important role in the initial ideas
about pranayama. Our ancients first came to see that for the
preservation of life we must preserve breath, and preserving
breath entails two things, i e., breathing slowly, and then not
breathing (for a short time) at all. This idea was further streng-
thened by the belief that the length of one's life is to be measured not in terms of days or years, but in terms of how many
times one is destined to breathe. From the fact that the stoppage
of breath and the end of one's life coincide, our ancients pro-

bably conceived the idea that when the number of breaths one was destined to take was exhausted, one could not live any longer. This idea is conveyed even today in phrases like 'breathing one's last,' for indicating death.

The idea that the breaths of everyone of us are numbered, that our life-span is dependent on how many times we shall breathe in a given life, and that, as a consequence of this fact, we must reduce the number of breaths so as to live longer—this idea was responsible for the origin of pranayama. We have this idea clearly mentioned at several places in the ancient texts on pranayama. For instance, it is declared in the *Gorakshapad-dhati* (I.93), that

"Due to fear of death even Brahma, the Lord of creation, keeps on practising pranayama, and so do many *yogis* and *munis*. Hence it is recommended that a student of yoga must always control his breath."

In the same manner the *Hathayoga-pradipika* (II.39) says,

"All the gods including Lord Brahma became devoted to the practice of pranayama because they were afraid of death. We the mortals should follow the same path and control the breath."

It may be that the origin of pranayama, as is clear from the above references, was influenced by the idea of conquering death through the control of breath. But later on many other advantages must also have come to light. We shall have occasion to consider them at a later stage.

Why do we breathe at all

Taking it for granted that breathing means living, and vice-versa, one may still wonder why life is so dependent on breathing, and why it comes to an end when breathing becomes impossible. All of us know that we cannot live without air. But very few of us are in a position to say why this is so. It would be very helpful to be aware of the processes involved in breathing in order to understand how pranayama can be used for the prevention and cure of disorders.

To begin with we must differentiate between breathing and respiration. In common usage these two terms are often used as synonyms. But actually respiration is a wider term. Breathing is

a physical or mechanical act performed with the help of specialised organs, in which air, or more specifically, oxygen from
the air enters the body, and then the air together with the im-
purities from the body such as Carbon dioxide and water
vapour, is drawn out of the body. Respiration, as a wider term,
includes this act as well as the further process of carrying the
absorbed oxygen to every part of the body and distribut-
ing it throughout the body. In case of man and higher
animals we may say that they breathe as well as respire. But in
case of plants, lower forms of life, and micro-organisms, there
is only respiration and no breathing, because there are no organs
for breathing. A new-born baby starts breathing just after
birth when the lungs are filled with air for the first time. Before
birth, in the womb of its mother it does not breathe, but respiration still exists, and oxygen is supplied to each cell of its growing
body inside the womb.

Now let us see why oxygen is indispensable for life. Every
living tissue and cell requires a constant supply of energy to
live. To be alive means to undergo certain bio-chemical processes. These processes which are the essence of life cannot go
on without energy. This energy is stored in the molecules of
certain substances such as glucose, fructose, fatty acids, and
amino acids. These molecules are the end products of the process of digestion of food materials which we eat. The energy
stored in these molecules can be released from them only
through a chemical interaction called oxidation of the energy
containing compounds, which cannot take place without oxygen. In the absence of oxygen the process of release of energy
comes to a halt, which means the death of that tissue. Oxygen
is already present in the atmosphere on earth. At sea level there
is about 20% oxygen in the air. This oxygen cannot be utilised
by the cells and tissues of our body directly from the atmosphere. It has to be carried to each cell and tissue. This important
job of carrying oxygen to each minute part of the body is done
for us by the blood. This is called internal respiration. The task
of bringing oxygen in contact with the blood is called external
respiration. It is the same thing as breathing. Thus breathing
may be called the outer expression of the process of internal
respiration. Thus if breathing stops, then each cell and tissue
of the body which requires oxygen continuously for keeping on

the process of oxidation in order to release energy stored in the end products of carbohydrates, fats, and proteins, would be starved of oxygen. Lack of oxygen means no further oxidation, which means no supply of energy for the bio-chemical process of living, and that inevitably results in the death of that cell or tissue. That is why life is solely dependent on breathing. This was perhaps the reason why our ancestors used the word prana both for the air we breathe and for the essence of life, namely, the soul. But even if it is true that breathing is so vital for life, one may still wonder whether there is any advantage in controlling the breath. That is our next question.

Why should we control the breath

It may be observed that whenever we are required to go into action at once, such as while taking a long or high jump, or lifting a heavy weight with all our might, or hitting a hard blow, and so on, we automatically stop the breath. Breathing is also arrested when there is a sudden shock and when there is complete absorption of the mind in something interesting. This shows the relation between intense physical or mental activity and breath control. This control is brought about by the nerve centres in us which govern breathing activity. In pranayama, we control the breathing activity by bringing into action inhibitory impulses from the brain. This point shall be discussed in greater detail later on. Here we are discussing why we should control the breath at all.

It is true that for carrying out various activities of daily life we do not have to control the breath at all. It is already being controlled and modified according to the needs of the body by the respiratory centre without our being aware of it. For instance, while we are resting, breathing automatically slows down, whereas, when there is physical activity necessitating an increased supply of oxygen and the faster removal of carbon dioxide, breathing automatically becomes faster and deeper. Thus controlling the breath is not required for the usual activities of daily life. Control of the breath is, however, undertaken for another reason, which is of interest to all of us.

It is one of the basic pre-suppositions of yoga that the breath (prana) and the mind (*chitta*) are not separate or inde-

pendent of each other. They are, in fact, considered to be two
different expressions of one single basic entity. They are interdependent. They work together and stop working together. We
are using both the entities, namely, breath and the mind constantly. Breath is important because our existence depends on
it. Mind is important because everything that is necessary for
success in life such as pleasure, happiness, enjoyment, our
relationship with the world, our reactions to the happenings in
and around us, are all dependent on it. If the mind is well
trained, peaceful, and full of contentment, that is to say, under
one's control, then life becomes fruitful.

This fact is brought out in a very clear fashion in the *Katha
Upanishad* (I.iii. 3 to 6) as follows:

"The soul is like a traveller who has set on a journey of life
in the chariot of the body, driven by the intellect (*buddhi*) with
the mind for the reins and the sense organs being the horses.
The objects of experience form the way to be traversed. The
soul, senses, and mind together form the enjoyer of pleasure
and pain, i.e., the individual. If the mind is not properly controlled, then the senses go out of hand like untrained horses.
But if the mind is properly controlled (*yukta*) then the senses
obey the orders of the master, i.e., the individual, like well
trained horses. Indeed, such an individual reaches the highest
goal of life."

Now to control the mind, howsoever essential it may be for
success in life, is one of the most difficult things to achieve. All
of us are aware that if we would control our minds we could
make life happier and far more enjoyable, both for us and for
others. Still we find ourselves helpless. It is here that pranayama
can come to our aid. The ancient masters of yoga knew that
even if it is very difficult to control the mind directly, it can be
controlled by controlling the breath. They mentioned this at
several places in the yoga texts. For instance, the *Yogavasistha*
(V. 78.46.) has explained:

"When through continued practice of pranayama the vibrations of breath are silenced, that causes the mind, too, to become
completely silent. That is the state of *Nirvana*."

This same point is brought out in the *Hathayoga-pradipika*
(IV. 23) by saying,

"Where the mind is absorbed completely, the breath also is
silenced, and vice versa."

The *Annapoornopanishad* has gone a step further to make
the point clear. It has emphasized (II.89) the oneness of mind
and breath, and so, has stressed the importance of pranayama
for controlling the mind thus:

"The vibrations of breath or air (*pavana*) are the same as
the vibrations of the mind. So the thoughtful attempt to control the vibrations of breath."

Many other statements from ancient texts can be quoted
here to show the significance of pranayama for silencing the
mind. But it is hardly necessary to multiply examples. The
whole point of view may be summarised in the following declara-
tion of the *Annapoornopanishad* (II. 44):

"Yogis control the breath in order to have peace of mind
(*chittashanti*)."

It may be said on this that all of us are not yogis, and so
pranayama is not useful for all of us. But that is not true, because every one of us needs peace of mind, and if it can be
achieved through the practice of pranayama, then pranayama
would certainly be useful for all of us.

This does not mean that peace of mind is the only end for
which pranayama is practised. In fact, it is a rather distant goal,
although it has been emphasized largely in the traditional outlook on pranayama. There are more easily achievable and
nearer goals, such as the maintenance and restoration of health,
efficient functioning of the various systems of the body, especially the respiratory system, and cure of disorders such as
asthma, hypertension, diabetes, and so on. These effects of pranayama will be discussed thoroughly in a further chapter.

What can pranayama do

It is essential for everyone interested in learning and practising pranayama to know what it can and cannot do. For
instance, it should be understood that not every disorder can be
treated by pranayama. Similarly, it is not equally useful to all of
us. There are certain conditions under which pranayama can-

not and should not be practised. It is also necessary to know
how pranayama works, so that all possible dangers in its practice
can be avoided.

A student who wants to learn pranayama and continue
practising it needs to have a clear idea regarding its scope and
limits. As a part of yoga, pranayama should normally be practised along with other parts, such as asanas and meditation.
This gives better results especially in the prevention or cure of
disorders. We shall discuss in detail the utility of pranayama in
relation to this in a later chapter. In the beginning it is helpful
to eliminate some false beliefs about pranayama which are common even among some yoga teachers. We shall consider these
beliefs in the chapter to follow.

2

Misconceptions About Pranayama Removed

It may appear strange that although yoga has become quite popular today, not all the techniques included in yoga have attracted equal attention. We hear a lot about yoga in general and hundreds of new books on yoga appear every year. But very little is said about pranayama. Compared to other parts of yoga such as asanas and meditation, the training and practice of pranayama is lagging behind. People who come to know about the usefulness of yoga as a curative measure often ask which asanas they should practise for overcoming their disorders. This is because in most of the training classes of yoga, in talks and in the literature on yoga, asanas are emphasised more than any other part of yoga. Most of our yoga experts are experts of asanas or of meditation. If one becomes aware of the importance of pranayama and seeks to learn its techniques it is hard to find a trained teacher. One is not usually encouraged to practise pranayama. This situation has resulted from many beliefs entertained by people about pranayama. Most of these beliefs are caused by ignorance. It is necessary to clear them in the very beginning. We shall consider them here one by one. Of course, not all these beliefs are totally false or wholly baseless. They do have some basis, and it is important to know the basic facts underlying them.

1. Pranayama is not for the householder

Until a few years ago, when yoga had not yet become popular, it used to be believed that to practise yoga one had to become an ascetic. This belief is not so strongly held now, but it is still argued that to practise the esoteric or higher parts of yoga, strict rules pertaining to food, sex life, and general conduct must be observed. Pranayama is considered one of the parts of yoga requiring strict rules of conduct. The common man is not supposed to be in a position to observe these rules strictly. Hence it is believed, by and large, that the common man should not indulge in the practice of pranayama.

If we analyse this belief in terms of its contributing factors then it would be found that there are two main reasons for holding this belief. First, in the ancient traditional writings pranayama is associated with things such as the arousal of the dormant kundalini power, the removal of the veil of ignorance that covers the mind, and the absorption of the mind in a state of silence. These are said to be the effects of pranayama. Since these are beyond the reach of the common man, the practice of pranayama has come to be believed as being beyond the abilities of many of us. But it should be understood that the effects the ancient texts have ascribed to pranayama in very high sounding terms are not the only effects it produces. For the maintenance of health and the cure of disorders, pranayama has tremendous implications. And these are within the reach of the common man. The ancient texts have emphasised mainly the effects of an intensive practice of pranayama. That is clearly not for the common man. But pranayama can be practised moderately in a small measure and for lesser or nearer goals. These goals, although not stressed in the traditional texts, are significant today. These goals can be attained without being an ascetic. What these goals are, and how they are achieved, are problems which we shall discuss in a later chapter. It is important to note here that there are nearer goals for pranayama and that they are within the reach of most of us.

Secondly, the belief that pranayama is not for most of us has arisen from the fact that no proper guidance is easily available. But this situation can be changed. There are already some signs of improvement in this direction, and the number of properly trained experts of pranayama is increasing.

So the belief that pranayama is not for the householder should be replaced by the statement "pranayama is for all of us, although the higher goals like kundalini-arousal, samadhi, and mukti may be beyond our reach."

22   YOGIC PRANAYAMA

2. Pranayama is dangerous, so its practice should be avoided as far as possible.

This is perhaps a more widespread belief and it is held more seriously compared to the first belief discussed above. There have been instances of people who have suffered mental and bodily disorders due to a careless and excessive practice of pranayama. But this should not mean that pranayama should always be shunned. Any instrument or technique which is used indiscriminately and without proper care may lead to dangerous results. That is true of almost everything, even of highly beneficial things such as medicines, exercise, food, virtues, love, and so on. The excessive and improper use of any good thing is dangerous. Pranayama is no exception. The danger involved in the practice of pranayama can be compared to the danger associated with crossing a crowded street, driving a car or handling a sharp instrument. If we observe traffic rules properly we can move quite safely on the streets. Millions of us do this daily. Those who work with elephants, lions, or tigers in a circus are always face to face with danger. But most of them still go through life merrily. Pranayama as an art of taming the prana or breath is compared to the taming of these beasts in the *Hathayoga-pradipika* (II. 15). Their training needs patience and care. Lack of patience and care may lead to the death of the trainer. Prana in pranayama may also act like a killer, says the text, in a similar manner, i.e., without proper care and patience. The text has brought out clearly the difference between properly practised (*yukta*) and carelessly practised (*ayukta*) pranayama (II. 16), and has declared that the former cures many diseases while the latter gives rise to many of them. This is a very important fact about pranayama. We shall elaborate it further while discussing the actual practice of pranayama.

Thus instead of saying that pranayama is dangerous, we should say that pranayama can be dangerous, and that its practice should be followed, not avoided, as far as possible, because there are many benefits which we get from it.

3. As pranayama is the fourth part in Patanjali's scheme of yoga, its practice should begin only after mastering the first three parts, namely, yama, niyama, and asana.

This is a view held by some yoga teachers. They argue that the eight parts of yoga mentioned by Patanjali are to be practised in sequence, mastering the yama and niyama first, then asanas, then pranayama, then pratyahara, and only then the *antarangas* such as dharana, dhyana, and samadhi. It is true that unless the first five parts of yoga are practised the mind cannot be stabilised in the state of dharana. The human mind which is unsteady by nature requires some training to make it steady. So the *bahirangas*, i.e., the first five parts, which provide the necessary training for the mind must be followed first, and only then can one practise the last three parts of Patanjali's yoga. But this does not mean that the eight parts are such that one cannot go to the second part unless the first is crossed, and so on.

Perhaps this confusion has its roots in the tendency to take Patanjali's eight-fold yoga as a ladder having eight rungs or as a path of which samadhi is the destination. When we follow a path to reach a place of destination then some places on the way are met with first, some others next to them, and so on upto the goal. Similarly, it is thought that yoga forms a path on which yama-niyamas come in the beginning, then asanas, then pranayama, and so on upto samadhi, and that this order is to be strictly followed and cannot be changed, just as the order of places on a path cannot be changed. Or just as in a ladder the steps are to be climbed one after the other in a fixed order, i.e., the lower rung first, then the next higher one, and so on, it is argued that pranayama being at the fourth place in the order, should be practiced only after the first three parts of yoga are mastered.

Regarding this belief it may be pointed out that it is true only in a general sense and that it may have some significance only for those who want to tread the path of yoga upto the state of samadhi. In a general sense the belief only indicates the fact that there is an intimate relation between the eight parts of yoga mentioned by Patanjali, and that each one of them is to be considered as a part of a whole, just as the individual parts of our body are parts of a whole. The parts would lose their significance if considered in isolation and out of the context of the whole. And this fact is of value for one who wants to reach the final goal of yoga, i.e., mukti. For one whose curiosity is limited, who is aware of his limited capacities, and who has set for himself the goal of using yoga as a means for the maintenance and restoration of health, it is not necessary to first study and practise the yama-niyamas and master the various asanas before undertaking to learn the techniques of pranayama.

By saying this we are not minimising the relative importance of any part of yoga: It is true, indeed, that all the eight parts of yoga are important even for the common man in daily life and that this importance should always be stressed. But it is true also that we need not ask a yoga enthusiast who wants to learn pranayama for a health problem to wait until the yama-niyamas and asanas are perfected. Some people hold extreme views in this regard and say that unless one has perfected the yama-niyamas one has no right to be called a yoga student for any purpose, and that unless one has perfected an asana and developed the capacity to sit in it for one or two hours one should not think of practising pranayama. Such extreme views are clearly incorrect. The correct attitude would be to look upon yoga and its parts as a means and not an end in itself, to recognise the importance and interconnection of them as parts of a whole, and to make use of one or more of them according to one's needs. Of course, the relation between pranayama and asana cannot wholly be overlooked because pranayama is always to be practised while sitting in a suitable asana. But perfecting that asana by being able to sit in it steadily and comfortably for hours is a different matter which has not much relevance to the practice of pranayama, for the common man.

4. Pranayama should be practised only after taking initiation or gurumantra from a spiritual teacher. Otherwise it becomes ineffective.

This belief is held by those who do not approve of practising pranayama only for health reasons. They are impressed more by the spiritual aspects of pranayama, which, according to them, must always be regarded as more important. But it is

unnecessary to quarrel with them, because if one attains physical benefits from the practice of pranayama, and there are
many such benefits as we shall see later, their significance can
not be denied, although from the point of view of the spiritually
minded such a person may be looked upon as being deprived
of the higher benefits. The vast majority of us are actually not
particularly interested in those higher benefits, although they
may be revered, and there may be a few persons who achieve
them.

Mantra is a useful thing and so is pranayama, and to combine them would be very desirable. But it must be remembered
that although they can be applied jointly with advantage, they
also have their own special domains.

5. Pranayama gives unusual powers.

This is one of the most widespread belief about pranayama
held equally by those who never practise it and by persons who
display miracles of yoga for earning money and popularity.
There are many such miracles displayed on occasions at different places. Until a few years ago yoga used to be identified
with these miracles, and those who displayed them often said
that they gained the miraculous powers from an intense practise
of pranayama. Now-a-days yoga is not so associated with
miracles because its common benefits are being increasingly
understood. But miracles still have a great influence on the
popular mind, and many of them are claimed to be attained
through pranayama.

On examination miracles often turn out to be frauds or
tricks. Some may be genuine but they are not usually allowed
to be put to a scientific scrutiny, and not much is known about
them. They have a strong appeal to the common man, who is
credulous. Learned men also contribute to them due to covert
vested interests. Among the miracles associated with pranayama
we may list unusual physical powers such as stopping a car,
passing a road roller on the chest, breaking metal plates or
glass or stones, stopping the pulse and remaining underground
in a pit for days or weeks. It is claimed that by holding the
breath one can generate tremendous power which by training
can be diverted to and concentrated in any part of the body. It

is also claimed that one can learn to live without air or oxygen by pranayama training. In addition some persons claim that by practising pranayama one can make the body so light that it can float in the air. This is called levitation. It is much talked about but not usually shown in public. The other miracles mentioned above are shown more commonly.

What is the truth about these miracles which many of us might have seen a number of times? To discard them as total humbug would be fanatical because we have actually seen performers stopping a car or coming out of a pit alive after many days, and so on. But it should be remembered that seeing a performance is one thing, ascribing particular meaning to what is seen, quite another. There may be a wide gap between what we see and what we take it to mean. For instance, the fact that a person came out of a pit after many days only means that he was alive there for that long a time. To say that since he was practising pranayama in the pit and stopped breathing, and perhaps, even stopped his heart, and so could live without air, would be a wholly unwarranted conclusion. To draw such a conclusion there must be more evidence about the state of being of that person while he was in the pit. Such information can be very well supplied by using instruments such as the pneumograph, Electrocardiogram, and even EEG to the person in the pit. Air samples from the pit can also be taken from time to time. That would indicate clearly whether one is breathing or not and whether the heart is functioning or otherwise. But this needs full co-operation from the performer. Such cooperation is not usually forthcoming, and that is a pity. The field of yoga is full of charlatans. Their strength lies in the credulousness of the masses. But with the application of scientific procedures to the techniques of yoga and pranayama, which has started all over the world, the truth about the miracles of pranayama and how they could best be utilised for the benefit of humanity, would be clear.

6. Pranayama nullifies the effect of heat or cold.

It is claimed that if one practises pranayama one is not troubled by the effects of heat and cold. In severe cold so much heat can be generated in the body that warm clothing is

unnecessary. In the summer heat, pranayama can be practised
to nullify its effect. In the ancient yoga texts, two different
varieties of pranayama, one for producing cold and another
having the opposite effect, are mentioned. The former is called
Shitali, and the latter Suryabhedana. It is said that there are
two currents flowing in our body. One is called *Chandra-nadi*.
It is associated with the left nostril. When it predominates
while breathing a cold effect is produced. The other current
called *Surya-nadi* is associated with the right nostril. Its pre-
dominance in breathing gives rise to heat in the body. By
adjusting the currents in pranayama one is supposed to be able
to produce the desired effect.

But these two varieties of pranayama have in fact not much
to do with body temperature. If the above claim was true then
it should have been observed that Shitali pranayama would cause
the body temperature to fall, while Suryabhedana pranayama
would result in a rise of the body temperature. But actually no
appreciable changes in the body temperature have been observed
in experiments with these two varieties of pranayama. The con-
cepts of Chandra and Surya have another significance which we
shall discuss later.

7. Pranayama gives the capacity to hold the breath infinitely.

A student of pranayama is often asked the question: How
long can you hold your breath? It is felt that by practising
pranayama, the duration for which one can hold the breath is
increased considerably and thus one can remain without breathing for a long time. In a single act of holding the breath an
average individual may record a time of nearly one minute or
more. This period, it is supposed, can be increased very largely
by the practice of pranayama. But this is not very true. In
pranayama it is not important how long one can stop breathing
in a single act of holding the breath. Pranayama actually avoids
such a thing. Holding the breath is an act which is preceded
and followed by inhalation and exhalation. And these two acts
called puraka and rechaka are also given due importance in
pranayama. How long one can hold the breath with deep and
prolonged inhalation and exhalation is what is more important
than how long one can hold it with a forced inhalation and

then gasping for breath after the retention. A fixed ratio of time is to be observed between the three acts of inhalation, retention, and exhalation. That is more important than merely holding the breath abruptly.

But the belief that pranayama gives the capacity to hold the breath infinitely is true in another sense. An intense and prolonged practice of pranayama gives rise to the state called kevala kumbhaka in which the breathing process automatically and effortlessly comes to a stop for a while when the mind is completely peaceful. This state is very different from the state of merely holding the breath.

8. By saving the breath in pranayama one can prolong one's life.

We have already mentioned this belief earlier. It may be true that a person practising pranayama regularly would have better chances for a long life. That is because pranayama involves training of the muscles and nerve centres related to the breathing process, thereby making them function in an efficient manner. In fact, every function of the body is influenced beneficially by pranayama, as we shall see later. This is what makes for a longer life. Just as a machine works longer and more efficiently if regular servicing is done, similarly, pranayama services the whole body and mind, and thus makes for a healthy long life.

9. Beliefs regarding relation of pranayama with food.

It is believed that a person practising pranayama must have good food, otherwise the practice would be harmful. There is also the belief that by doing pranayama one can develop a capacity to remain without food for a long time. Pranayama is called Vayubhakshana, i.e., eating the air, and one who has mastered this art is supposed to draw the nutrition required for the body and mind from this, thus making the eating of food unnecessary. It is also believed that by practising pranayama one can digest any kind of food. Such beliefs are not true in their extreme forms, although in a general way they do have a a vestige of truth. For instance, good food is necessary for all of us including those who practise pranayama. The problem of food suitable for a student of yoga is important, and so we shall be discussing it separately in detail.

The argument regarding going without food seems to be based on the supposition that from the food we eat we ultimately get what is called *'pranashakti'*, or the source of energy which is essential for sustaining life. It is believed that this energy can be directly imbibed by doing pranayama, and so it is immaterial whether one eats food or not. Such a belief is not in keeping with the scientific knowledge of our times.

About the power of digestion it may be pointed out that even some ancient texts do speak about digesting poison and overcoming hunger and thirst through the practice of pranayama. (see *Hathayogapradipika* II. 57) But this, indeed, is not for the common man.

We have so far considered a few commonly held beliefs in order to remove possible confusion regarding what we can reasonably except from a practice of pranayama. It is not our intention to show that all these are false beliefs. But it is necessary to understand them in the right perspective before one actually starts pranayama.

We shall now see in the next two chapters how one should actually proceed to practise the various techniques associated with pranayama. First the preliminary conditions before making a start shall be discussed, and then the techniques themselves will be described.

3

Before Making A Beginning

From what we have discussed so far it is clear that prana-yama is a skill which can be acquired only through proper training and practice. It may be called an art of breathing to our best advantage. It is also a science of breathing which explains those advantages and tells us what takes place through the practice of pranayama, in our body and mind. After becoming aware of the usefulness of this art or science through reading a book or by visiting a yoga class, when one decides to learn and practise pranayama, some questions arise at the very beginning. There are three reasons for which one usually turns to pranayama. It may be done as a part of exercises to keep fit. Or there may be a health problem for the solution of which one is advised to take to its practice. It is a happy sign that more and more physicians and consultants are becoming aware of the importance of pranayama for the prevention and cure of certain ailments. There are some persons who practise pranayama as a part of spiritual *sadhana*, but their number is very small.

We shall consider here the initial steps to be taken for preparing oneself for pranayama before making an actual start.

Proper arrangements for training

For learning any technique or art it is very important to have an experienced teacher. Books can provide useful know-ledge about most things. But when something is actually to be done or practised, the knowledge obtained from books is not enough. For example, if one wants to learn to drive a car or to swim or paint or play a musical instrument, it is essential to get instructions from someone who is experienced in doing these things, who knows the do's and dont's of the practice, whose information is reliable, and who has some interest in teaching.

A few years ago it was not easy to get a good experienced teacher of pranayama. But this did not pose much of a problem as the number of inquiring students also used to be extremely small. Now with the growth of interest in pranayama the number of trained teachers has also increased, although much remains to be desired regarding arrangements for training. While there are many institutions and training centres, a common standard regarding the norms and procedures is not yet evolved. Those who have succeeded in collecting enough followers and money want to make it their own affair. They show little regard for others in the field. It is rather strange to see that the established yoga teachers often show a tendency to go alone, to try to emphasise an individual or his family or institution, and to strive to make a mark by inventing special brand names for some techniques and coining new phrases and names for themselves. Just a cursory look at any issue of the many periodicals concerning yoga may show very clearly the excessive concern of these individuals with the projection of their own images, their own ideas, likes and dislikes. Such a thing is not seen in the case of the established sciences such as medicine, physics, engineering and psychology. In the case of these sciences an individual's opinion as such has little importance, and what really matters is whether there is any impartial verifiable evidence that would support any particular opinion. But in yoga the situation is very different. Here every opinion, idea, or belief is highly personalised. The established yoga teachers have a vested interest in it.

This situation will change as more and more scientifically trained persons get attracted to the field of yoga in general and pranayama in particular. It is very essential for developing pranayama as an impersonal universally applicable science, that people should give up the immature attitude to strengthen the egoistic and monopolistic tendencies of the so called gurus, by following them blindly, and learn to depend on more verifiable evidence rather than high sounding inventions.

But it is difficult for a student to know who is a good teacher and who is not in the beginning. Those who talk too much, who always abuse others, or are too harsh and superficial do not make good yoga teachers. Similarly, those who want money and cheap popularity should be avoided. A good yoga teacher is moderate in his approach, ready to listen to others, and never extravagant in his claims. A humble, considerate, well educated gentleman conscious of his own limitations and having a good background of scientific training would make a good yoga teacher. Exact knowledge of the traditional texts, and capacity to explain the underlying facts involved, are two essential qualities of a good yoga teacher. He would have faith in yoga but not blind faith, and an interest in conveying what he knows to the student without bringing in his own ego. Those who talk much about themselves or their guru must be shunned. One must be considered lucky to have a wise and knowledgeable teacher for pranayama, because such teachers are not very common.

Fitness of the student

We have said so much about the teacher for pranayama. But what about the student? What qualities should a student of pranayama have? Is everyone fit to practise pranayama? These are some of the questions a student of pranayama should ask himself.

Regarding the qualities of a student it should be said that the minimum expectations from a student of pranayama would depend on what his purpose is, i.e., on how far he wants to go in the practice. For one who wants to practise pranayama as a part of spiritual sadhana with the aim of attaining samadhi or arousing the kundalini power or something similar, a deep sincere interest, inquisiveness, patience, and capacity for rigourous work would be essential. Celibacy, control of diet, and strict disciplining of the body and mind would be required. But most of the students of pranayama would not be interested in all this, as they may not have the time and the will to go very far in the practice of pranayama. As we have pointed out earlier most of us take to the practice of pranayama for the maintenance or restoration of health. For that purpose the above qualities are not a must.

But any student of pranayama, whether with a limited or deep interest, must have the will to learn the techniques and the basic facts. The purpose and the interest may be limited but not the sincerity and the will to understand. Clarity of understanding is necessary for all students. A casual approach would not produce good results. Persons suffering from a disorder such as asthma or diabetes which is amenable to pranayama, start with great enthusiasm and interest, but later the enthusiasm fades away and they become irregular in practice. This should not happen. Half heartedness does not yield good results.

While learning pranayama for the first time it is better to start the practice when one is in a normal state of health. If the health is impaired or if one is convalescing or very weak, then it is better to postpone the first lessons till one recovers completely. This also holds good when pranayama is to be begun with a view to overcome some ailment. For instance, as a curative measure for asthma, pranayama should not be begun when the attack is on. Pranayama is an exercise of a special kind. Like other types of exercise it also requires that one should not exert oneself in a state of illness. If one is too tired after physical or mental exertion, then pranayama should be done after resting. Similarly, after tiring physical exercise like swimming or wrestling one should rest and then do pranayama. In the same way, pranayama should not be practised while one is feeling too hungry, or soon after taking meals. If one is awake for a long time and feeling sleepy, then it is better to postpone the pranayama session until one is refreshed again.

The question is often asked whether it is essential to take a bath before doing pranayama. In the minds of many of us a bath is associated with religious observances, and pranayama is very much akin to religious observances. But actually there is no connection between the two. It is true that after taking a bath one's mind becomes fresh and the body clean. This is good for pranayama, but it is not a must.

In short, while doing pranayama one should be in a normal state, and if this condition is fulfilled then almost everyone of us is a fit person for practising pranayama.

Age for starting pranayama

Like any other art pranayama can be enjoyed throughout life. But what is the best age to learn it? A general answer to this question is: the earlier the better. At the age of eight or ten years deep breathing in a moderate measure may be started. But holding of breath should be postponed upto the age of fourteen. Adults may start doing pranayama at any age, there being no upper age limit for making a start. Pranayama provides one of the best preventive means for disease such as asthma, arthritis, diabetes, and disorders of the digestive tract. Those who are prone to such disorders should learn to do pranayama as early as possible so as to get the best results. Even as a curative technique it is good- to take the earliest possible opportunity to start doing pranayama so as to give it a fair trial. The saying 'better late than never' is very true about pranayama, and it is always useful to remember it.

For both the sexes

Pranayama is equally useful for men and women. Or it may be said that it is even more useful to women than men, because compared to men women lag behind in taking regular exercise. Their activities are mostly indoors and they have much less physical exertion. So women are more prone to suffer from the lack of exercise. Exercise of the abdomen and pelvis is far more important for women than for men. Pranayama exercises these parts, helps to remove congestion of blood, and tones up the muscles. Thus it has a great therapeutic value for disorders concerning menstruation, position of the uterus and natural child birth.

If a woman understands the importance of something and starts practising it then everyone in the house is influenced by the beneficial effects of it. Training housewives in the art and science of pranayama would thus have a great additional advantage for the spread of pranayama among all members of society.

Surroundings and selection of the place

Ancient texts abound in reference to the selection of a suitable place and surroundings for the practice of esoteric yoga including pranayama and dhyana. Although that has no relevance for most of us in the present times, it would be interesting to know what our ancient texts recommended. It is recommended that a student should stay in a province with a stable government, ruled by a kind, religiously minded ruler and inhabited by religious masses. There should be no fear of invasion and no disturbance from beasts, thieves, bad characters, insects, epidemics, and natural calamities like draught or floods. One is advised to stay under the direct supervision of a guru in a secluded place, absorbing pleasant surroundings, where all the needs of food, shelter and peace of mind are well taken care of.

Some of these needs would be felt even by the present day students of pranayama. For instance, one must have for practising pranayama a peaceful, clean, airy place where there is enough privacy and the least of disturbance due to noise, visitors, and other factors. The best place for the modern student would be the home, if the above needs can be fulfilled. Sometimes one may enjoy practising pranayama at a peaceful place on the bank of a river, or in a park or temple.

In big cities where homes are small and usually crowded, pranayama may better be practised in groups in big rooms or halls belonging to educational or other institutions, specially engaged for that purpose. But practising pranayama individually at home is to be preferred wherever possible. Even in the beginning when one learns it in a class it should be learnt individually.

After the techniques are learnt properly and one is sufficiently practised in the art, it is immaterial whether the daily practice is performed in a class room or at one's home, in the office or outdoors. While on a journey even a train carriage or an aircraft with a comfortable seat may be considered good enough for practising pranayama.

What to wear while doing pranayama

This would depend on the climate, social norms, individual liking, and preferences. While practising pranayama in the open, the clothing should be sufficient to protect the body from cold. In pleasant weather especially while practising in a room just an underwear may suffice. In hot weather a short or loin cloth may be all that is necessary. The clothes should cover the body neither too much nor too scantily. There should be no feeling of discomfort due to tight or too many clothes while one sits in an asana for some time during pranayama. While practising in groups in classes a common uniform may be desirable.

Time of practice and length of a sitting

For ordinary purposes pranayama may be practised once a day either in the morning or evening. In the evening after a day's work the mind is relaxed and the muscles and joints are not stiff because they are worked up during various movements of daily life. So one finds it a bit easier to assume a posture for pranayama and to hold it steady for the required length of time. In the morning the joints are rather stiff but they can be made more amenable by some warming up exercise. In the evening one may have visitors or one may have to go out for social calls and for household duties such as marketing. In the morning there is usually less disturbance due to these causes, and so from the point of view of regularity the morning is a better time.

There is another consideration which makes the morning more suitable for the practice of pranayama. It is an important requirement that while practising pranayama the stomach must not be loaded. There are considerable changes of internal pressure inside the thoracic and abdominal cavities taking place with each round of pranayama. A loaded stomach would interfere with these changes of pressure. In the morning before having breakfast the stomach is already empty. In the evening this may not be the case and that may cause irregularities in the practice. For having an empty stomach one should allow two hours to go after breakfast and four hours after a meal.

After a cup of tea about an hour should pass, before one gets ready for pranayama.

The length of a sitting would depend upon how much pranayama one is practising. Ordinarily about twenty minutes would be quite sufficient. On very busy days, if there is too much work one may have a ten minute sitting rather than going without a pranayama session.

Diet and food habits

Is it necessary for a student of pranayama to be a vegetarian? This is a question asked quite seriously by those who come to learn pranayama. There is no set answer to this question. The answers given by teachers show a wide range. On the one hand there are those who say that the student of pranayama should give up even taking tea or coffee, not to speak of eating meat or fish. At the other extreme there are some modern gurus who would say that no restriction on diet or sex life is at all necessary. The truth seems to lie midway between these two extremes.

The problem about diet divides itself into two parts: what to eat, and what not to eat. Regarding the latter part, there is a wide variation of opinions as mentioned above. About the former part there is uniformity, and it is said that the diet of a student of pranayama should be *sattvik*. According to yoga philosophy, everything in the universe shows a mixture of three basic tendencies called *gunas* in varying proportions. These three gunas are respectively called *sattvaguna*, *rajoguna* and *tamoguna*. Sattvaguna stands for lightness, cleanliness, brightness, pleasure, happiness, understanding, knowledge, peace, justice, and so on. Rajoguna represents activity, unsteadiness, excitement, envy, anger, obstacles and the like. Tamoguna manifests itself in the form of heaviness, inertia, laziness, lack of drive, pain, darkness, and ignorance. All items of food are divided into three groups. Some are sattvik, having a preponderance of sattvaguna. Some are *rajasik*, i.e., having more of rajoguna. And those which give rise to effects characterised by tamoguna are called *tamasik* foods. In the Bhagavadgita we have a detailed description of these three gunas and their manifestations. Some of the items of sattvik food are: cow's

milk, melted butter, rice, barley, honey, sweet fruits, coconut,
dates, and some vegetables such as soft gourd. Sattvik food is
supposed to give rise to sattvik effects. A student of pranayama is advised to take only sattvik food. Meat, fish, eggs,
wine, onions, garlic, spices, and chillies are considered rajasik.
Hence they should not form a part of the diet of a sattvik
person.

This view about yogic diet, which has been held traditionally on a very large scale may be true in a very general sense.
Perhaps it is true only in a few extreme cases. Actually there
is no intimate relation between what one eats and what one
thinks or does. Otherwise it would be possible to change all
the criminals in jails to good respectable persons simply by
feeding them on sattvik food.

The question of vegetarianism has two aspects, one dieteti-
cal and the other emotional or ethical. Those who advocate
vegetarianism often fail to distinguish between these two
aspects of the question. This has given rise to some confusion
about the problem. It is very important to note that the dieteti-
cal considerations of the problem are different from the ethical
considerations. Of course, a solution which is both dietetically
and ethically sound would be the best. But there is no such
single solution which would be useful for all persons, because
the nutritional requirements of different persons vary to a large
extent. It is no good to prescribe the same kind of diet to
growing children, convalescents, nursing mothers, athletes,
officegoers, and those people who do heavy work, using their
muscles. Students of pranayama may belong to all these
different groups. To say that they should all eat only sattvik
and strictly vegetarian food would set an unnecessarily rigid
standard. When the ancient texts prescribed such a standard it
was meant for those who had left their jobs and homes for the
sake of devoting their life solely to a deep study of pranayama
and dhyana. The ancient texts did not err in their prescription
of diet, but we shall certainly be committing an error if we
apply those prescriptions to all of us in a wholesale manner.
Most of us who take to the practice of pranayama have to play
our roles also in the family and society.

Ethically the question is not what we should or should not
eat, but whether we should kill for the sake of food. This is not

a question for the dietician to decide. It is to be decided on what ethical standards we want to follow. Surely, there cannot be a set standard in this regard for all persons and for all times. Such a standard can be prescribed for the advanced students of pranayama, as has been done by the ancient texts. But that may not be applicable to all of us. This much about a sattvik diet and vegetarianism.

An average student of pranayama may still wonder as to what should be the best diet for him. There is a very useful piece of advice on diet in the *Hathayoga-pradipika* (I. 63) for all of us. It lays stress on what is called *mitahara* or balanced diet, and says, "The diet should contain all the necessary nutrients, should be tasty, should have enough milk and milk products, and it should supply nourishment to all the constituents of the body. One should like to eat it. Above all, it should be conducive to the purpose on hand." This last qualification for which the text uses the word '*yogya*', meaning fit, useful, or justified, would allow a variety of items of food, vegetarian or otherwise, depending on the role one has to play in life.

A few general hints on diet may be given here. It is always a good policy to avoid eating or drinking those things which cause disturbance to or which do not suit one's system. What is good for one may not be good for another. Overeating should always be avoided. Eating too many times is a vice. What we think and do is more important than what we eat or what we do not. Not taking wine or flesh or even tea or coffee has no value as such in itself. It is very important to include raw uncooked vegetables such as carrots, radish, onion, cabbage, cucumber and similar items, as well as sprouted seeds (raw or cooked) in the diet. Fruits and milk form the most likable and useful items of diet. The diet should supply enough calories but not an excess of them. The use of fried items should be limited. It may not be necessary to give up any particular item but the excess of anything must always be avoided. Occasional fasting, liquid diet, and missing a meal once in a week or fortnight are very useful things for health. These hints are for people having normal health. In the treatment of disorders diet is to be more carefully regulated.

Combination of pranayama with other activities

Pranayama is a respiratory exercise. One may be doing other kinds of exercise also, and it is not necessary for the student of pranayama to give up other exercises. If that exercise involves much physical activity as outdoor games, running, jogging, swimming, and sun prostrations called Surya-namaskara which is one of the popular exercises in India, then pranayama should be done after that exercise, allowing at least ten minutes to lapse in between, so that the process of respiration comes to normal. Pranayama consists of taking deep and slow breaths and retention of breath. So it should never be combined with any rigorous physical activity which necessitates rapid breathing. In quick forceful activity one automatically holds the breath momentarily, e.g., while lifting or throwing a heavy thing or while jumping. But that is not an example of doing pranayama.

Many students of pranayama may be practising asanas also, along with other exercises of a rigorous type. In such a case the more active exercise should be done first, then asanas, and then pranayama. If dhyana or meditation is practised, it should follow pranayama, as pranayama prepares the body and mind for meditation. Taking a walk for a mild exercise may either precede or follow pranayama. While walking or doing asanas the breath should not usually be controlled deliberately. So pranayama should not be mixed up with other exercises although it may be combined with them in the above sequence.

Regularity of practice

Pranayama, like any other art can produce pleasant results only with regular practice. Many persons who take it rather casually do it regularly for a short time in the beginning, and then irregularity creeps in. Then there may be a long gap during which the benefit, if any, is lost, and then the practice may ultimately come to a halt. If one has realised the need and understood the importance of pranayama then it has to be made a part of the daily routine. Yet there may be gaps in the practice due to exigencies of work, travel or illness. For overcoming these one should have a firmness of mind and a kind of faith and devotion. Laziness is often a major cause of irregularity. Lack of patience is another factor to be avoided. When there is a gap due to any unavoidable reason it should be remembered that one must resume the practice at the earliest opportunity. If one is doing pranayama alone at home then more strength of mind is required to overcome the interfering factors. If one has joined a class or a group then the influence of others helps to keep on regular practice.

Although practising pranayama seven days a week and thirty days a month would be ideal, it is not very essential ordinarily to be so regular. Taking one holiday every week does not interfere in any way with the benefits. Two offs in a week may be all right if it happens occasionally and not too often. It is a useful general policy to decide that one shall not miss a pranayama session unless there is some unavoidable reason for doing so. One should always try to have a session rather than going without it by curtailing the duration if necessary.

Measurement of time

Normally in a resting condition we breathe in and out without noticing the fact that we are doing so, nearly fifteen times every minute, taking a little less than two seconds for each inhalation and slightly more than two seconds for each exhalation. In pranayama this duration of each round of breathing is increased, filling and emptying the lungs as completely as possible in each round. A definite proportion of time is to be maintained for the three acts of inhaling, holding, and exhaling which comprise each round of pranayama. For this an exact measurement of time in seconds becomes necessary. The ancient masters of yoga prescribed different mantras for this purpose. A mantra is a string of words to be repeated again and again with a uniform speed of utterance. It serves two purposes: first, the form of prayer or the meaning of the words of the mantra helps the mind to become peaceful. Secondly, when one learns to recite the mantra uniformly it provides a means to measure time. The famous Gayatri mantra is specially suited here, because it consists of three parts which can be employed during each one of the three stages of a round of pranayama. But that is good for an advanced student, not for a beginner.

A beginner may better use a stop watch for measuring time. Or a wrist watch with a clear dial and a centre second may be used. Here the student has to pay attention to two things simultaneously, that is, the breath and the watch. This is not very difficult, but some students do find it a bit confusing. For them a table time piece is better. It makes a fixed number of sounds, usually one hundred per minute. Keeping the time piece nearby and counting the sounds one can adjust the counts for inhalation, exhalation, and retention in each round of pranayama. Here one does not have to look at a watch, but still there are two things requiring simultaneous attention, namely, breathing and counting. If this is found difficult then a metronome which sounds a bell after a specified passage of time may be used with advantage.

Whatever the means employed, exact measurement of time in seconds should be possible without difficulty, because each round of pranayama has to be completed in equal time.

A clear nasal passage : Neti

It is not possible to practise pranayama unless the nose is clear. The passage in both the nostrils must be open. There should be no choking. It is essential to have a uniform controlled flow of air during inhalation and exhalation. It is observed that usually both the nostrils do not flow equally, one having a clearer passage than the other. This normal inequality of flow does not offer any problem for doing pranayama, because the difference is slight. If a nostril is partially clogged then breathing through it becomes uneasy and troubled. And if it is completely clogged then it cannot be used for breathing at all. There are many ways in which a partially or completely closed nostril can be opened up for the flow of air. These are discussed in a branch of yoga called *svara-shastra*. For instance, if the left nostril is choked it can be opened by lying down on the right side for some time, by pressing a ball or a stick called *yogadanda* in the right armpit, or by leaning to the left in a standing position and putting pressure on the left foot. For opening the right nostril these techniques are to be followed on the opposite side.

Persons suffering from chronic cold, sinusitis, or asthma often have one or both the nostrils closed. When they want to practise pranayama for a cure of these disorders a problem arises. They cannot do pranayama unless the nasal passage is cleared. For them there is a technique called *neti* which may be used with advantage. It is one of the six cleansing techniques of yoga called *shuddhikriyas*. Neti is of two types: *jalaneti* and *sutraneti*. The former is easier but less effective. In it *jala* i.e., water is used for cleansing the nose from inside. Water is taken in a pot specially meant for the purpose. The pot has a spout which is inserted in one nostril. The head is tilted on the opposite side and slightly forward so that water can be poured through the nostril. It comes out through the other nostril. One can learn this technique just in a day. No effort is to be made to suck water or to force it out. The water should be lukewarm, not hot or cold. A teaspoonful of common salt is added to one pot of water (about 300 ml. of water) so that it does not irritate the mucous membrane and acts as a better cleansing agent. After it is emptied one should blow the nose, fill the pot again, and pour water through the other nostril. This cleanses the nasal passage.

But if one or both the nostrils are choked completely then jalaneti is not possible. In that case one may try sutraneti. Sutra means a thread. Actually the sutra for neti is made of eight or ten pieces of soft cotton yarn, about 40 cm. in length. Along half of this length another thin fine soft yarn is wound up so that this end can be inserted in one nostril after lubricating it with butter or oil, turning it and pushing it slowly in. About two inches from the tip of the nose the nasal passage curves backward and downward and to insert the end of the sutra down this curvature without causing friction and irritation some care is to be taken. This can be learned by experience. After passing this curvature the sutra goes easily upto the throat. Then the student should open the mouth, pass the thumb and the index finger of the hand in and slowly pull the end of sutra out. Then both the ends of the sutra are held in the two hands between the thumb and the index finger, and are pulled alternatingly, so that the sutra rubs against the nasal passage and cleanses it. Sutra neti is far more effective than jalaneti for cleansing the nasal passage. After cleansing one nostril the sutra is pulled out through the mouth, washed, lubricated again, and inserted in the other nostril, repeating the whole procedure once again.

Apart from providing a clear nasal passage necessary for pranayama, neti helps to overcome the above disorders.

Preparing the seat

As mentioned earlier, to practise pranayama one has to assume a sitting posture first and maintain it steadily and effortlessly throughout the session. One may sit on the floor or on a bed or table. A comfortable seat is required. This may be about three feet in length and breadth. If there is a carpet or rug spread on the floor one may put on it a small carpet or blanket folded to make a seat of the required size and cover it over with a clean piece of cloth which can be washed frequently. The seat need not be too thick and soft. A piece of foam cushion can be used. If one sits on a bed no padding may be necessary. The seat should be such that one does not feel the hardness of the floor or surface of the table or bed. One should enjoy sitting. Deer hide or tiger skin is traditionally preferred because it does not allow heat or cold to pass through and it has a very soft feel.

Whatever the material used for preparing the seat, one should see that it offers a plain surface without sagging and allows one to hold an erect sitting posture comfortably.

Postures suitable for pranayama

Why should we not do pranayama in a standing position or while walking or doing some work or lying down? Every student of pranayama should know the right answer to this question. When there is any physical activity in the body involving repeated contractions of muscles, more energy is expended for the work done as compared to a resting state, and the oxidation process in tissues is increased for the supply of energy. This necessitates more oxygen intake, and therefore breathing automatically becomes rapid. This is the opposite of what we do in pranayama. Thus it is clear that pranayama and muscular activity should not go together. It is always necessary to have a resting state of the body while doing pranayama. One may ask here whether it is not the case that while doing pranayama we imbibe more oxygen as compared to normal breathing. This is a belief entertained by many of us and even by some yoga teachers who have not received proper training. But the fact is otherwise. We shall explain this point in detail while discussing the effects of pranayama.

It may be argued that if only a resting body is what pranayama requires, then in a lying down position we fulfil this condition best. Regarding this point it is important to note that pranayama involves controlled movements of the muscles of the chest, back, neck, and abdomen. A lying down position interferes with that and so it is to be avoided.

One important characteristic feature of the sitting postures recommended for pranayama is that in them the body is held erect, allowing free movement of all the parts associated with respiration. These are called meditative or meditational postures, because they are the most useful for practising meditation. They are the best suited for pranayama also. A good practice of pranayama very easily leads to a state of mind necessary for meditation. There are four such postures traditionally available. If one is unable to practise any one of them, which is sometimes the case, then a posture called Sukhasana may be assumed. This should be done only in exceptional cases. We shall describe this posture first and then the four traditional ones.

SUKHASANA

Sukha means pleasure. Sukhasana is a posture in which one can sit with pleasure, i.e., without a feeling of discomfort. Actually, every posture when mastered well becomes a sukhasana. This is explicitly stated by Patanjali in his definition of a posture where he uses the word 'sukha' as a necessary quality of a posture. Sukhasana means sitting cross-legged with an erect back and neck. Many people find even this difficult, especially those who have stiff joints. But with a little practice one can sit comfortably in a squatting position as required in sukhasana. This is the easiest of the sitting postures. When the sukhasana becomes easy, one should learn one of the other four traditional postures, because they are more advantageous.

In one of the ancient texts (*Darshanopanishad*, III. 12.) Sukhasana is described thus:

"In whatever sitting position one may attain comfort and steadiness, that is called Sukhasana. It is to be assumed by the weak."

VAJRASANA

Vajra means lightning. It is the name of the weapon of Lord Indra of Hindu mythology. Hardness is its outstanding quality. In Hathayoga and Tantra the word vajra is used for the male sex organ. Vajrasana is a sitting posture in which the thighs are arranged in the form of a vajra. This is said in the *Gheranda Samhita* (II. 12). The feet are kept behind the hips with the soles turned upward, heels apart, and toes of both sides touching each other. One sits between the heels and not on them. The knees are kept together in front, the shins touching the floor. The back should be kept erect. Keeping the feet in the position described above is very uncomfortable in the beginning especially if the surface of the floor is hard. So there should be enough thickness and softness in the seat prepared for sitting in this posture. It should not be done on the bare floor. With a few days' practice one starts enjoying it. This is somewhat akin to the posture in which devout Muslims sit for their Namaz prayer.

SWASTIKASANA

Swasti means welfare. It is a word to express one's approbation. *Swastika* is a symbol denoting good luck. It also means crossing the arms or making a sign like the cross. Swastikasana is a posture in which the legs cross each other below the knees and the toes are placed in the inner hollow of the knees, thus imitating the figure of a swastika.

For doing swastikasana the student should first sit on the seat cross-legged and set the right heel against the left groin, putting the toes between the left thigh and calf. The left foot is then set in the same fashion on the right side. The legs should cross each other a little above the ankle. Both the knees should rest well on the seat. The hands are kept on the knees. One should sit erect without stooping or pulling the shoulders back.

Holding the back and neck straight, the body should be held in
a relaxed state without there being any stretch or strain. We
find a description of this posture in most of the important yoga
texts. The above is a summary of that description.

SIDDHASANA

This is somewhat like Swastikasana in appearance, but
more strenuous. A novice may not easily be able to tell the
difference between the two by seeing their pictures. But the
difference is crucial.

Siddhi means achievement. In yoga it usually means mystic
supernatural power. A *siddha* is a person having such powers,
or one who has become an adept. Siddhasana is the favourite
posture of the siddhas or the posture which gives siddhis. It is
considered to be the foremost among the postures of yoga. All
major texts have spoken about its importance in high terms.

For assuming Siddhasana, the left heel is set against the
perineum, i.e., the space between the anus and the genital organ,
placing the right heel over the left one. The knees must be well
placed on that seat. The toes are to set between the calf and
thigh on the opposite side. Thus this posture differs in the place-
ment of heels from Swastikasana. In the latter the heels are
placed on the two sides of the genital organ in the same horizontal plane, while in Siddhasana they are in the same vertical
plane with the genital organ, the left one below and the right
one above it. In Siddhasana there is more stretch on the legs.
The pressure on the perineum and genital organ by the two heels
is a special feature of this posture. This, together with the increased stretch on the lower back or rather the tip of the spine
plays an important part in arousing the Kundalini power. That
is why this posture enjoys the most superior position among all
the yoga postures.

In some yoga texts this posture is called Vajrasana. For
instance, in the *Yogakundali Upanishad* (I. 6) we find the
technique of this posture described under the name of Vajrasana. One is asked to sit with a straight back, neck and head
with the left heel below the penis and right one above it. In
some texts the right heel is said to be put below and the left one
above. (see *Jnaneshwari* commentary of the Bhagavadgita, VI.

194,199). This would provide an answer to a question often arising in the minds of students practising the meditational postures, namely, whether we can change the position of the legs or if one particular foot is always to be kept below and the other one above. It seems that the tradition would allow both the alternatives available. This applies equally to Swastikasana, Siiddhasana, and the next posture called the lotus pose that we are going to describe immediately.

PADMASANA

Padma means a lotus. Another word denoting a lotus is Kamala. So Padmasana is sometimes also called Kamalasana. The significance of this name is that in this pose one imitates the figure of a blooming lotus. Many ancient idols of Lord Buddha and Lord Mahavira are found to be seated in this pose or the Siddhasana pose. The appearance of the lotus is imitated with the feet and the hands.

The student sits on the seat with the legs in front. The right foot is held with the hands near the ankle and is placed on the left thigh with the sole turned up and the shin touching the thigh. The left foot is then similarly arranged on the right thigh so that both the heels nearly touch each other. Both the knees should be kept on the seat. Keeping the back and neck erect, the hands are placed on the heels with the palms facing up, the left hand below the right one. The thumbs and fingers should overlap each other to give an appearance of the petals of a lotus, the feet imitating two leaves. Many students and yoga teachers are not aware of this fact concerning the significance of the name 'Padmasana.' So they keep the hands on the knees. In many books we find a picture of Padmasana given that way. While assuming the posture for the purpose of pranayama, however, one hand would be used for closing one or both the nostrils. But while practising meditation the hands must be kept on the heels as described above.

Padmasana is a widely described posture. Its full form as a meditative posture includes two more techniques, namely-gazing at the tip of the nose and fixing the chin below the throat. In traditional terminology these are respectively called *Nasagra drishti* and *Jalandhara bandha*. Similarly, the full form of Sid-

Postures Suitable for Pranayama

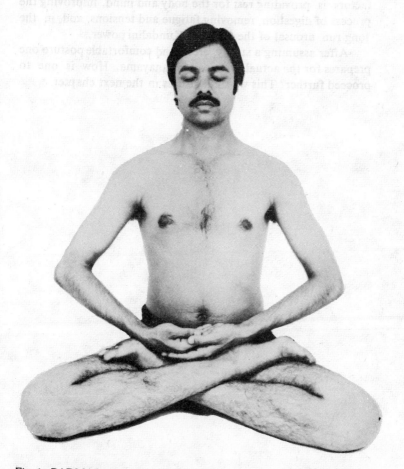

Fig. 1 : PADMASANA : Keep the right foot on the left thigh and left foot on the right thigh. Keep the hands on the heels.

dhasana includes gazing between the eyebrows, called *Bhrumadhya drishti* and also Jalandhara bandha. But while doing pranayama these two additional techniques are not to be followed.

These postures, whether they are practised in association with meditation or pranayama, involve folding, pressing, and stretching of the lower limbs, thus reducing the blood supply to them. More blood is supplied to the lower back. An upward pull is exerted on the spine and the wall of the abdomen. A state of deep relaxation is achieved. The combined effect of all these factors is providing rest for the body and mind, improving the process of digestion, removing fatigue and tensions, and, in the long run, arousal of the dormant Kundalini power.

After assuming a steady, erect, and comfortable posture one prepares for the actual practice of pranayama. How is one to proceed further? This we shall discuss in the next chapter.

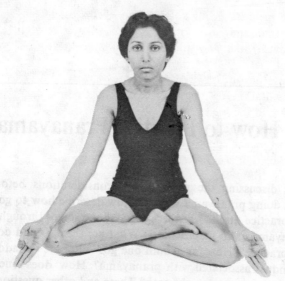

Fig. 2 : **SIDDHASANA** : Sit with the left heel set against the perineum and the right heel on the left one.

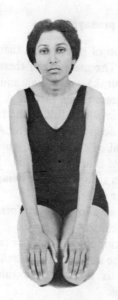

Fig. 3 : **VAJRASANA** : Sit between the heels, the greater toes nearly touching each other.

4

How to Practise Pranayama

After discussing the preliminary considerations before one starts doing pranayama we shall now describe how to go about the practice itself. Are there any definite stages through which pranayama is to be practised? What are the do's and dont's of the practice? How far should one go? What are the additional techniques associated with pranayama? How does one know that one is on the right path? These and other questions arise when one actually makes a beginning. Let us discuss these questions one by one.

Three components of pranayama

In any discussion of pranayama there are three oft repeated technical terms. The meaning of these should be very clear. These terms are: puraka, rechaka, and kumbhaka. We have already referred to these terms earlier. A puraka in pranayama is the act of inhalation which fulfills the following conditions.

(a) It should be deep and complete. At the end of a puraka the lungs should be filled completely, there being full expansion of all the parts of the lungs.

(b) It should be a slow act, there being no extra force applied for sucking the air in.

(c) The flow of air should be uniform from the beginning to the end of a puraka.

(d) The time taken by each puraka in successive rounds of a sitting should be the same. Thus puraka is not just any form of inhalation but it is a controlled inhalation fulfilling the above four conditions.

Similarly, rechaka is not just exhalation. It means a controlled exhalation which is slow, deep, uniform, and comp-

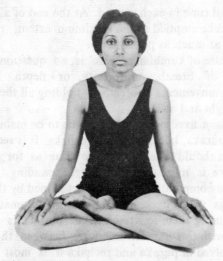

Fig. 4 : SWASTIKASANA : Sit with the feet crossing each other above the ankles.

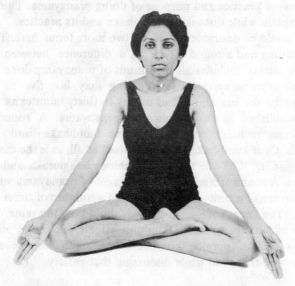

Fig. 5 : SUKHASANA : Sit at ease with a straight back, one foot under the opposite thigh and the other under the opposite leg.

leted in equal time in each round. At the end of a rechaka the lungs should be emptied to the maximum extent, their tissues contracting as much as possible.

In the case of kumbhaka there is no question of speed, movement of breath, uniformity, or depth. It involves stopping all movements of breath by holding all the respiratory apparatus tight and still.

There is a fixed proportion of time to be maintained with regard to puraka, kumbhaka and rechaka. It is recommended that rechaka should take double the time as for puraka. In puraka there is muscular effort for expanding the lungs. Rechaka is a comparatively passive act helped by the elasticity of the lungs which causes them to shrink automatically when the force causing them to stretch as in puraka is withdrawn. In keeping with this natural difference between the muscular activity involved in puraka and rechaka it is most convenient to give puraka half the time as for rechaka. Some yoga teachers advocate equal time for them, but giving double time for rechaka is much better.

How long one should do kumbhaka depends upon the progress of practice and purpose of doing pranayama. This we shall explain while discussing kumbhaka and its practice.

It would be desirable to clarify two more terms here. They are: a sitting and a round. There is a difference between the two. A sitting includes all the rounds of pranayama done one after the other in succession. A sitting may last five to ten minutes in the beginning, and twenty to thirty minutes as one gets established in the practice of pranayama. A round of pranayama includes one puraka, one kumbhaka and one rechaka. Or if kumbhaka is not practised at all, as is the case in the beginning, then one round will include one puraka and one rechaka. A round includes all those stages of pranayama which together make a unit which is repeated a number of times in a sitting. The length of each round should be the same. In a variety of pranayama called Anuloma-viloma one round includes two each of puraka, kumbhaka and rechaka. We shall explain why that is so while discussing that variety.

Three Components of Pranayama

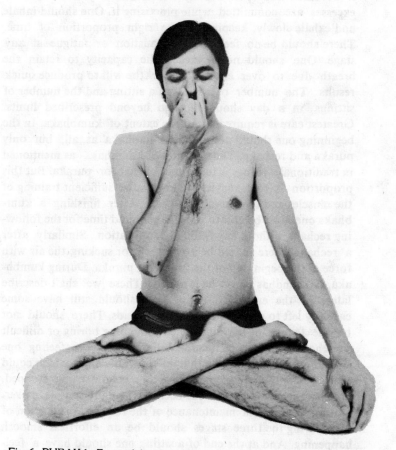

Fig. 6 : PURAKA : Expand the chest fully and uniformly, without allowing the abdominal wall to bulge.

Yukta pranayama

It has been mentioned earlier that pranayama if practised
properly can help us to overcome many disorders and if practised in an improper manner it can give rise to disorders, sometimes of a serious nature. In this context it is important to
know the essential characteristics of *yukta* pranayama and how
it becomes improper. Pranayama is called yukta when no
excesses are committed while practising it. One should inhale
and exhale slowly, keeping to the right proportion of time.
There should be no feeling of exhaustion or fatigue at any
stage. One should never exceed the capacity to retain the
breath due to over enthusiasm or the will to produce quick
results. The number of rounds in a sitting and the number of
sittings in a day should not go beyond prescribed limits.
Greatest care is required about the extent of kumbhaka. In the
beginning one should not practise kumbhaka at all, but only
puraka and rechaka. The duration of kumbhaka as mentioned
in traditional writings is four times of that for puraka. But this
proportion is to be achieved slowly after sufficient training of
the muscles and the nervous centres. After finishing a kumbhaka one must be able to give the required time for the following rechaka without any feeling of suffocation. Similarly, after
a rechaka there should be no craving for sucking the air with
force at the beginning of the following puraka. During kumbhaka, the bandhas must be applied. These we shall describe
later. At the end of a sitting one should still have some
capacity left to undergo a few more rounds. There should not
be the feeling of having finished something boring or difficult
somehow and that one is now relieved. But the feeling one
should experience must be that an enjoyable affair which could
easily be continued for some more time is now being stopped,
not because one is tired but because the daily routine is over.
During pranayama maintenance of the required proportion of
time during the three stages should be an effortless smooth
happening. And at the end of a sitting one should have a feeling of peace and satisfaction. These are the requirements of
yukta pranayama.

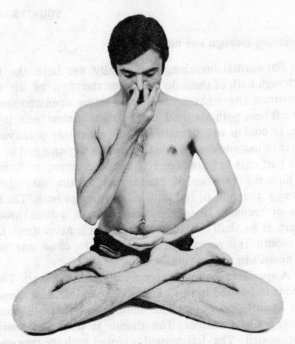

Fig. 7 : KUMBHAKA : Hold the breath in after puraka, without straining the respiratory apparatus.

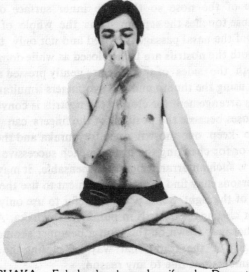

Fig. 8 : RECHAKA : Exhale deeply and uniformly. Do not bend the shoulders.

Breathing through one nostril

For normal breathing we usually use both the nostrils. Although both of them do not allow the flow of air equally, sometimes the right nostril being more open and sometimes the left one, both are used in breathing unless one is choked due to cold or other reasons. While practising pranayama it is better to use one nostril at a time in the beginning. The nostrils take part only in puraka or rechaka, but never in kumbhaka. In different varieties of pranayama puraka may be done through the left or right nostril or through both. The same is true of rechaka. In some varieties puraka is done through the mouth as we shall see later. But rechaka is never done through the mouth. It is necessary to learn how to close one or both the nostrils in pranayama.

A special technique is recommended in the texts. The right hand is to be used in this. The index and middle fingers are bent against the palm. The thumb and the two remaining fingers are kept straight. The thumb is used for closing the right nostril. The left nostril is closed with the ring and little fingers. Closing of a nostril is to be effected not by closing the aperture but by pressing the thumb or the fingers gently on the side of the nose so that the inner surface of the side of the nose touches the septum. Thus the whole of the front portion of the nasal passage is closed and not only the orifice. When both the nostrils are to be closed as while doing kumbhaka, both the sides of the nose are gently pressed against the septum, using the thumb and the two fingers simultaneously.

This arrangement for closing the nostrils is convenient for all purposes because the position of the fingers can be shifted easily to keep one nostril open for puraka and the other for rechaka or for changing the order in each successive round.

But is such an arrangement indispensable, it may be asked. Some persons may find it more convenient to use the left hand in place of the right. Some persons prefer to use only the index finger for closing the nostrils in puraka or rechaka. A traditional teacher may frown on this. But a beginner should be given some laxity if the traditional way of closing the nostrils is found cumbersome due to any reason.

Varieties of Pranayama

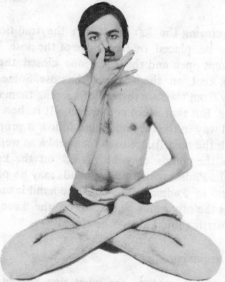

Fig. 9 : ANULOMA-VILOMA : Breathe in and out through alternate nostrils, taking deep, uniform breaths.

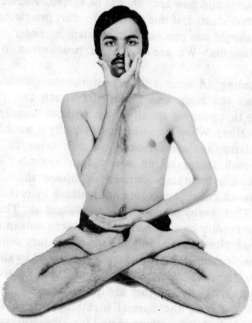

Fig. 10 : SURYABHEDANA : Use the right nostril for puraka and the left one for rechaka in each round.

While closing the left nostril in the traditional way the thumb is to be placed on the bridge of the nose. When the left nostril is kept open and the right one closed the two fingers are to be kept on the bridge of the nose. Some persons hold them away from the face instead of keeping them on the bridge of the nose. But that is not convenient. It is best to learn the traditional way in the beginning and follow it properly.

If both the nostrils are used for puraka as well as rechaka, then both the hands may be placed on the knees. If one is sitting in the Padmasana pose the hands may be placed on the heels. Even in Padmasana when one hand is used for closing the nostrils the other may be placed on the knee. In kumbhaka the nostrils should always be closed.

Making a beginning

We have discussed to far what one should know about pranayama before actually making a start, what the problems are that arise and how they should be solved. Remembering all the points discussed, if one wishes to start practising pranayama how should one proceed step by step in order to get the desired benefits? We are now in a position to discuss this problem.

Assuming an erect sitting posture one should close the eyes, relax the body and mind, and watch the process of breathing that goes on in all of us without usually catching our attention. When one watches it silently it would be found that inhalation and exhalation follow each other in successive rounds, each found taking nearly four seconds. Thus every minute we are breathing fourteen or fifteen times. To some extent we can change this rate of breathing by making it rapid or slow. That is why pranayama is possible at all. This capacity of ours to modify breathing at will is taken advantage of in pranayama. Normally in daily life the respiratory centres bring about modifications in breathing as required by the needs of the body. In pranayama the activity of these centres is controlled systematically and they are trained in a set pattern.

After watching the normal breathing process for a while one finds that while breathing in and out the full capacity of the lungs for expansion and contraction is not utilised. To fill

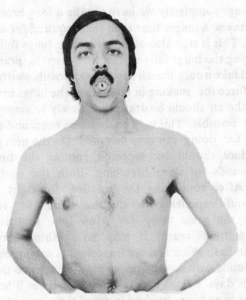

Fig. 11 : SHITALI : Do puraka by sucking the air in slowly through a channel-like arrangement of the tongue.

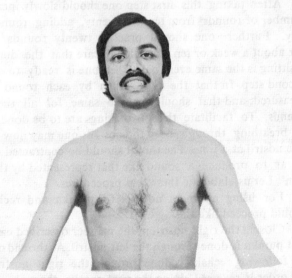

Fig. 12 : SITKARI : Breathe in through the mouth, along the surface of the tongue.

the lungs completely we have to take a long breath. This naturally takes a longer time than that required for a normal inhalation. This is true also of emptying the lungs fully. Filling and emptying the lungs fully is the first step in pranayama. One should take a deep breath as slowly as possible without using any extra force for sucking in air. When the lungs are filled completely the air should be drawn out slowly to empty the lungs as far as possible. This may be done ten times and the total time taken for doing this may be noted. On the next day the same procedure should be repeated, noting the time taken for ten rounds of deep breathing. Both the nostrils may be used. After continuing the practice for eight to ten days one should experience that the time taken for ten rounds is nearly the same every day. How long that time is, is not what matters much. It may be anything between two to five minutes. What is more important is taking equal time for ten rounds each day. Some people may achieve this in just two or three days. Others may take a longer time. When it is found that ten rounds are finished in equal time, every time it can be said that one has taken the first step in pranayama successfully by achieving uniformity in breathing.

After taking this first step one should slowly increase the number of rounds from ten to twenty, adding rounds every day. Further one should practise twenty rounds per day for about a week or ten days, taking care that the duration of a sitting is the same every day. Then one is ready to take the second step. In that the time taken by each round is to be measured, and that should be the same for all the twenty rounds. To facilitate this, two things are to be done. Instead of breathing through both the nostrils one may now use only one nostril at a time. The throat should be contracted slightly, so as to produce a sound like that represented by the letters 'hm' Let us elaborate these two procedures.

For using alternate nostrils for puraka and rechaka one should proceed like this:

Closing the right nostril in the manner described earlier, the first puraka is done through the left nostril. At the end of puraka the following rechaka is done through the right nostril. Then the order is reversed, doing the next puraka through the right and rechaka through the left nostril. This makes one round.

The Bandhas (Holds)

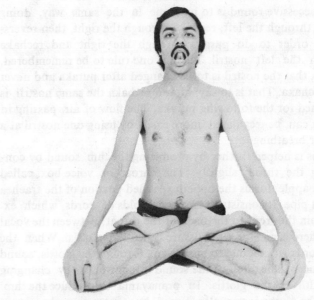

Fig. 13 : JIVHA-BANDHA : Keep the tongue tightly pressed against the roof of the mouth.

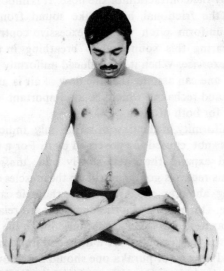

Fig. 14 : JALANDHARA BANDHA : Set the chin below the throat while holding the breath in.

Each successive round is to be done in the same way, doing
puraka through the left, rechaka through the right, then revers-
ing the order to do puraka through the right and rechaka
through the left nostril. There is one rule to be remembered,
namely, that the nostril is to be changed after puraka and never
after rechaka. That is to say, after a rechaka the same nostril is
to be used for the following puraka. The flow of air passing in
and out can be regulated more easily by using one nostril at a
time for breathing.

This is helped further by producing the 'hm' sound by contracting the throat slightly. The throat or voice box, called
Adam's apple, forms the upper expanded portion of the trachea
or wind pipe. It consists of two vocal folds or cords which extend from the front to the back of the throat. Between the vocal
cords there is an elongated fissure called the glottis. When the
vocal cords vibrate due to air passing through the glottis, sound
is produced. The pitch of the sound is controlled by changing
the width of the glottis. In pranayama to produce the 'hm'
sound the glottis is partially closed by contracting the throat
muscles, thus offering a slight resistance to the flow of air which
gives rise to the sound. This sound is different from the one
produced by the contraction of the nose. It is important to learn
to produce the frictional hissing-like sound from the throat
in a low uniform pitch without excessive contraction of the
throat. Hearing this sound while breathing in and out is an
absorbing exercise. When it is produced uniformly without ups
and downs one can assume that the flow of air is uniform during puraka and rechaka, which is an important condition to
be fulfilled for both of them.

But uniformity of the flow of air is only indicated by the
sound. It is not caused or governed by it. For a uniform flow
one should expand the chest slowly and uniformly during
puraka. This requires good control on the muscles of respiration
which bring about an expansion of the thoracic cavity by their
contraction. During rechaka these muscles are relaxed. A controlled relaxation of them synchronised with the elastic recoil
of the lungs is very essential for a deep and uniform rechaka.

Toward the end of puraka one should not allow the abdominal wall to bulge. On the contrary it should be slightly
tightened and pulled back by contracting the abdominal muscl-

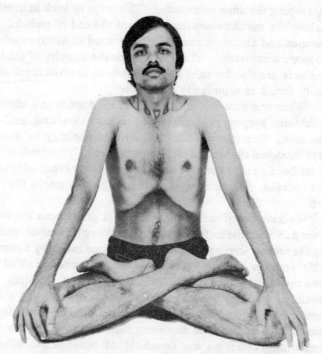

Fig. 15 : **UDDIYANA BANDHA** : After exhaling deeply, the chest is expanded without allowing the air to enter the lungs. This pulls the diaphragm upward in the thoracic cavity, pulling back the abdominal wall.

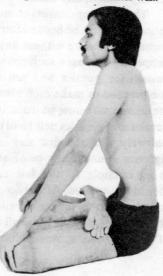

Fig. 16 : Side View

es, keeping the anus contracted. This helps to suck in more air making the puraka complete. Toward the end of rechaka also the anus and abdomen should be contracted so as to expel the air more completely. While doing this the muscles of the back and neck are also brought into action so as to make the thoracic cavity shrink as completely as possible.

When one succeeds in finishing all the rounds in a sitting in equal time, keeping the puraka and rechaka slow and uniform, and doing them through alternate nostrils, one may be said to have mastered the second step of pranayama. No attention had so far been paid to the proportional time to be given to puraka and rechaka. To start paying attention to that marks the third step.

We have noted earlier that puraka in pranayama should be given half the time as for rechaka. For doing this after mastering the second step one should note the time taken by a comfortable rechaka in two or three successive rounds. Half of that time should be given to puraka. When this is decided, one should go on doing twenty rounds in which each puraka will be completed in equal time and each rechaka will be done in double that time. When one can do twenty such rounds smoothly and comfortably one is on the threshold of pranayama. Whether one takes one or two or three months to reach there is immaterial. What matters more is that one should arrive there systematically without any haste.

The next step consists of increasing the time or length of each round. This can be begun after one practises twenty rounds of a particular measure without any difficulty for a fortnight or more. Supposing that each such round is of fifteen seconds, i.e., five seconds for puraka and ten seconds for rechaka, how should one proceed to make each round longer? From a fifteen second round one may now go to a twentyone second round in which puraka and rechaka will be of seven and fourteen seconds respectively. On the first day out of the twenty rounds the first eighteen rounds may be of shorter length, i.e., fifteen seconds in our example. In the last two rounds the longer duration should be applied. After two or three days the last four rounds may be of the longer duration. Proceeding slowly like this in about twenty days or more all the rounds in a sitting will be of twenty one seconds, duration. If there is a feeling of

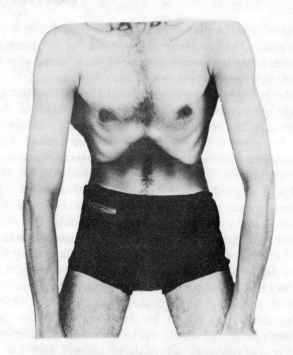

Fig. 17 : UDDIYANA IN STANDING.

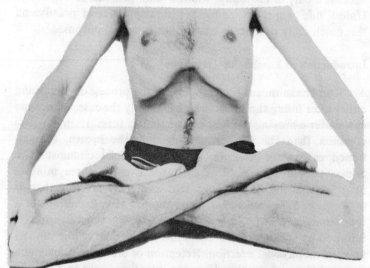

Fig. 18 : UDDIYANA SHOWING DETAILS: The abdominal wall assumes a concave appearance.

discomfort or suffocation at any stage one should halt the increase in practice and continue what one is doing for some more
time, attempting to increase the time of each round after more
practice. One should never exceed one's capacity.

After practising twenty rounds of the longer duration for a
fortnight one can increase it further, say, to a round of twenty
four seconds. The procedure is the same. After practising that
round for about a month one may take up a round of thirty
seconds which would include puraka for ten seconds and rechaka
for twenty seconds. Twenty such rounds would take ten minutes. This is a good measure of deep breathing which is quite
sufficient for daily practice for the maintenance of good health
and even in many cases as a therapeutic measure. For ordinary
purposes kumbhaka is not necessary at all. Some persons may
find it difficult to reach this stage even after a practice for six
months. Some may achieve it in just one or two months, and
some may find it quite comfortable to start their practice with
puraka of ten seconds and rechaka of twenty seconds. Individual differences in this regard are considerable. So one should
know one's limits and should not transgress them. After reaching the goal of twenty rounds of thirty seconds each one may
make it a part of his daily routine and practise it regularly.
Unless one wants to go further in the practice of pranayama
this much daily practice is enough for practical purposes.

Introduction of kumbhaka (retention)

Kumbhaka means the stoppage of the process of breathing
either after filling the lungs, which is mostly the case, or in some
cases after emptying the lungs. The latter form is much less
common than the former. We do hold the breath, as mentioned earlier, for brief moments under special circumstances.
Some people can do this even for two to three minutes
at a time as in the case of the pearl divers. But that is
not repeated in successive respirations. After retention for a
long time one may go out of breath and so the retention is
followed by taking rapid breaths just as one does while under-
going great physical exertion. Retention of breath in pranayama
is very different from this. Here the intention is not to hold the
breath once only or for the longest possible period, until one

Vastra Dhauti

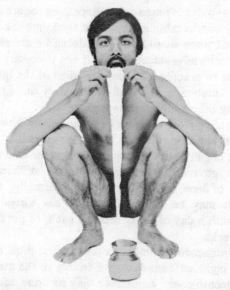

Fig. 19 & 20 : A process of cleansing the stomach by swallowing a strip of cloth moistened with water. One end of the strip must always be kept out of the mouth, so that the dhauti can be taken out after cleansing the stomach.

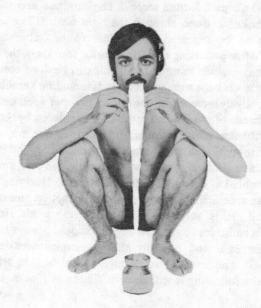

gets out of breath. Getting out of breath at any stage is to be
completely avoided in pranayama. Repeating the act in successive
rounds very comfortably is important for kumbhaka.

How and when should one start doing kumbhakas? Does it
have any special advantage? Why is it not necessary for ordinary purposes to practise it? These are some of the questions that
arise about kumbhaka. We shall discuss only the first of them
here, leaving others for later chapters.

As is evident from what we have said about how one should
go about for beginning the practice of pranayama, kumbhaka
is not to be begun until the respiratory system and the nervous
centres that govern its working are trained sufficiently in the
mechanism of deep, uniform breathing. Normally, as mentioned earlier, it may be begun after one has already practised
twenty rounds a day of thirty seconds each, of puraka-rechaka
for some weeks.

While introducing kumbhaka for the first time one should
go through eighteen rounds out of twenty in the usual manner.
In the nineteenth round kumbhaka may be done after puraka,
taking the same time as for puraka, i.e., ten seconds. Both the
nostrils are to be closed during kumbhaka. And the bandhas
should also be applied. These will be described presently. After
holding the breath for ten seconds the bandhas are withdrawn
and rechaka is done through the right nostril. The same procedure is to be repeated in the last round, alternating the
nostrils. After practising this for three or four days, the last four
rounds may include kumbhaka. If this can be done comfortably
then after a week the number of rounds including kumbhaka may
be progressively increased at the rate of two per week until all the
twenty rounds of puraka and rechaka are replaced by those including kumbhaka. If this is found difficult then one may continue
to practise only ten plus ten rounds excluding and including
kumbhaka respectively for some more time and then proceed to
have kumbhaka slowly in all the rounds. Hurrying towards
something spectacular without sufficient practice, must always
be avoided. It is very important to remember this. How much
practice is sufficient to proceed further should always be decided by the ease and comfort that one experiences during the
practice. If one exceeds one's capacity for holding the breath
the rechaka following it will show it. There will be a tendency

Jala Neti

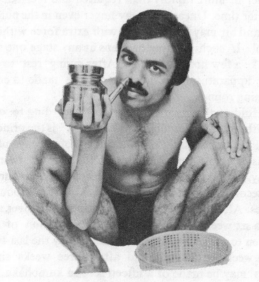

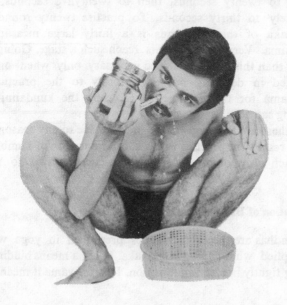

Fig. 21 & 22 : A process of cleansing the nasal passage by pouring lukewarm water through one nostril. The water comes out through the other nostril.

to expel air more rapidly than required and rechaka will end in
a shorter time. Uneasiness may linger even in the puraka following it and air may be sucked in with extra force without proper
control. If such a thing happens at any stage one should stop
and take a few normal breaths. After giving rest to the respiratory apparatus a fresh start may be made to complete the
remaining rounds.

"Holding the breath comfortably according to one's capacity without ever exceeding this capacity," is the principle which
should not be lost sight of by a student of pranayama. Following this principle, one should reach the goal of twenty rounds
per day, taking one's own time to reach it. Each round will take
forty seconds and a sitting will be over in about fourteen
minutes. After one practises such sittings daily over a period of
four to six weeks, one can increase the duration of kumbhaka
from ten to fifteen seconds. On the first day the last two rounds,
after a week four rounds, and after three weeks six or eight
rounds may be made of a fifteen second kumbhaka. This number may then be increased to twenty in due course, never
ignoring the case of performance. After one is established firmly
in the practice of kumbhaka for fifteen seconds, this time may
be increased progressively in the same manner as described
above, to twenty seconds, then to twentyfive seconds, and
ultimately to thirty seconds. To practise twenty rounds of
kumbhaka of thirty seconds is a fairly large measure of
pranayama. Very few students reach such a stage. Going still
further than this may be deemed necessary only when one is
interested in devoting oneself seriously to the practice of
pranayama for the purpose of arousing the kundalini and
attaining samadhi.

If there are long gaps in the practice due to any reason one
should restart the practice with a shorter duration of kumbhaka
and reach where one had left the practice in two to three
weeks.

Application of Bandhas (holds)

Bandhas are special techniques prescribed in yoga which
are applied while doing kumbhaka. Bandha means binding or
holding tightly in a certain position. In pranayama it means the

Sutra Neti

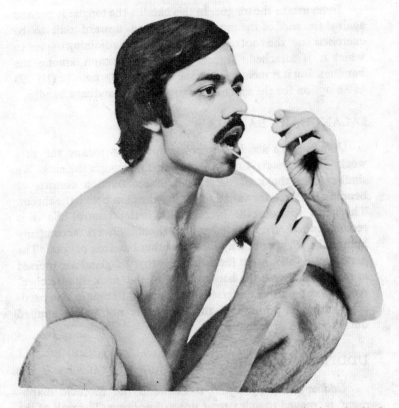

Fig. 23 : The sutra can be prepared by intertwining six to eight threads of soft cotton yarn. A rubber catheter can also be used. This process also cleanses the nasal passage by putting it through one nostril and taking out from the other. It is the foremost among the cleansing processes.

contraction of particular muscles of the body. There are four
main bandhas associated with pranayama. They are: Uddiyana
bandha, Jalandhara bandha, Mula bandha, and Jihva bandha.
We shall describe their technique and significance one by one.
Let us take the last one first.

JIVHA BANDHA

Jivha means the tongue. In this bandha the tongue is pressed
against the roof of the mouth causing an upward pull to be
exercised on the root of the tongue and the adjoining tissues to
which it is attached. This is the least common among the
bandhas. But it is mentioned in the *Hathayoga-pradipika* (III. 22)
as an option for the much more prevalent Jalandhara bandha.

JALANDHARA BANDHA

Jala means a net. In the present context it means the net-
work of the *nadis* or channels passing through the neck. We
shall explain the *nadis* later. Jalandhara bandha consists of
bending the neck forward and setting the chin below the throat.
This helps to hold the breath with better control. So it is
recommended that this bandha should always accompany
kumbhaka whether one applies the other bandhas or not. The
parts around the throat including the thyroid gland are pressed
in this bandha, and the back portion of the neck is stretched.
An upward pull is exercised on the spine. Except in one particular variety of pranayama, this bandha is not to be applied
during puraka or rechaka.

UDDIYANA BANDHA

Uddina means a jump. In this bandha the thoracic diaphragm is moved to an extreme upward position. The wall of the
abdomen is pulled towards the back giving a concave appearance
like the bottom surface of a pond. A pond is called *tadaga* in
Sanskrit, and this bandha is also called Tadagi Mudra in yoga
texts. That is done after an exhalation so that the depression in
the wall of the abdomen looks quite pronounced. When it is
done while holding the breath in, during pranayama the con-

Nauli

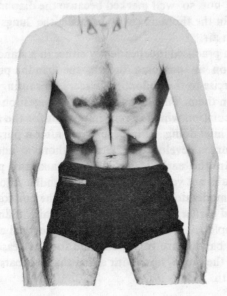

Fig. 24 & 25 : NAULI IN STANDING : This is better done in a standing position. It involves rotation of the abdominal recti.

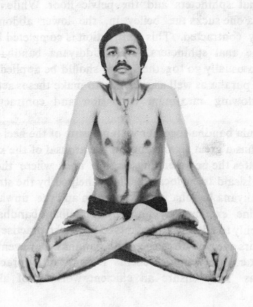

cavity is not so well marked because the diaphragm does not rise high in the thoracic cavity because the lungs are already filled with air.

When practised independently either in a standing or sitting position on an outgoing breath, the bandha provides a very good exercise to the abdominal viscera by causing pressure and stretch on them. This helps to remove congestion and promote blood circulation which is very important for the health of any organ. While doing it in pranayama after a puraka, a stretch and pressure is developed in both the thoracic and abdominal cavities. In the early stages of the pranayama practice when kumbhaka is not yet introduced, this bandha should only be practised moderately toward the end of the puraka. This, as we have noted earlier, helps to inhale more air, filling the lungs more completely. The physical and therapeutical advantages of Uddiyana bandha are very great, and for this reason it is compared in the yoga texts with a lion that combats the elephant called death.

MULA BANDHA

Mula means the root. Mula bandha is the contraction of the anal sphincters and the pelvic floor. While in Uddiyana bandha one sucks the belley in, the lower abdomen is also slightly contracted. This contraction is completed by contracting the anal sphincters. Thus Uddiyana bandha and Mula bandha usually go together. They should be applied toward the end of puraka as well as rechaka, to make these acts complete by allowing maximum expansion and contraction of the lungs.

Mula bandha together with pressure of the heel on the perineum has a great significance in the arousal of the kundalini. It stimulates the nerve endings in that area where the kundalini power is said to be located. This is helped by the stretch caused by Uddiyana bandha in the abdomen and the upward pull on the spine exercised by it and by Jalandhara bandha. That is of value only to advanced students of yoga who practise pranayama for hours everyday together with bandhas. But even an average student can draw many benefits from a little practice of the bandhas. They ensure an efficient working of almost every

Kunjal

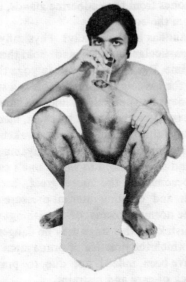

Fig. 26 & 27 : Also called Vamana Dhauti. After drinking lots of water, it is expelled from the mouth by a vomiting-like action.

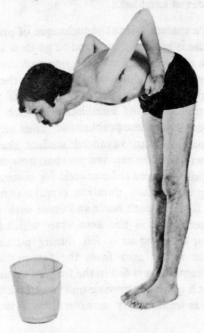

function in the body such as digestion, blood circulation, secretion of harmones from the endocrine glands, excretion of waste materials from the body, etc.

What do the bandhas bind actually? Physically they may be said to bind particular muscles and hold them tightly in position for some time. But that is not all. In yoga the bandhas are applied mainly for binding the prana. This is a special purpose for which pranayama is practised, and the bandhas help it greatly. The prana is said to be bound by them, made to have an impact on the kundalini, causing it to be awakened.

It should be remembered that when pranayama is practised along with the bandhas, the need to watch one's capacity and never to exceed it becomes all the more great, because while holding the breath and creating internal pressure and stretch one is modifying the normal process of breathing very considerably. A slight mistake at this stage may be dangerous. There have been cases in which the practice of pranayama has lead to disorders. These have been, indeed, not due to pranayama as such, but due to lack of care and restraint.

Three grades of kumbhaka

When a student learns the technique of pranayama for the first time he is naturally expected to go slow and continues the practice on a low note. But after one achieves expertise how much pranayama should one practise? Is there any final limit for the number of sittings per day, number of rounds per sitting, and the length of kumbhaka in each round? We have already considered these problems so far as an ordinary student is concerned. For an advanced student the answers to these questions will be different, and we shall now discuss them.

Patanjali has given three criteria for measuring pranayama, namely, space (*desha*), duration (*kala*) and number of rounds (*sankhya*). Space is both outer and inner with reference to the body. Outer space is the area upto which the impact of the incoming or outgoing air is felt during puraka and rechaka. Inner space is the area from the feet to the head where the impact of kumbhaka is felt in the form of sensations like those of the touch of an ant moving on the surface of the body. The duration was traditionally measured by a unit called matra.

Nasagra Drishti

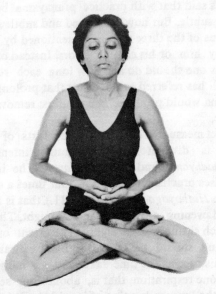

Fig. 28 : Involves fixing the gaze on the tip of the nose. Helps to arrest the movement of the mind and concentrate it.

Bhrumadhya Drishti

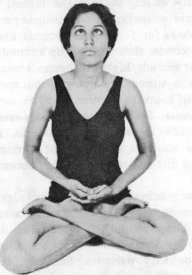

Fig. 29 : The eyes are fixed at the mid-point of the eyebrows.

Various measures of a matra are mentioned in ancient texts. Patanjali has said that with practice pranayama becomes prolonged and subtle. But how prolonged and subtle it should become in terms of the three measures mentioned by him, is not explained by him or his commentators. Instead of saying how many rounds one should do and how long each round should be, Patanjali has referred to the result that prolonged and subtle pranayama would produce. The result is: removal of the veil of ignorance.

The exact measure is described in the texts of Hathayoga. Pranayama is divided into three grades, intense (*uttama*), moderate (*madhyama*) and lowest (*adhama*). The intense measure comprises practising pranayama four times a day, as mentioned in the *Hathayoga-pradipika* (II. 11.), that is to say, in the morning and evening, at mid day and midnight. The number of rounds in each sitting is to be eighty. The extent of kumbhaka in each round should be twelve and half matras. A matra is defined in this case as the time taken by an individual while sleeping for one respiration, that is, about four seconds. This means that the longest duration of kumbhaka in intense pranayama will be about fifty seconds. Considering the ratio of time for puraka, kumbhaka and rechaka, which is one, four and two units respectively, we may say that the highest measure of a round of intense pranayama would include puraka for twelve seconds, kumbhaka for forty eight seconds and rechaka for twenty four seconds, thus making up a round of one minute and twenty four seconds. Eighty such rounds would mean nearly two hours for a sitting, and one may thus spend eight hours (seven and a half hours, to be more exact) per day in the practice of pranayama. Such intense practice is said to lead to the arousal of kundalini in six to twelve months. It is for such highly devoted students of yoga that selection of a suitable place, control of diet and rules of conduct become all the more important.

Moderate or madhyama pranayama includes kumbhaka of thirty two seconds, while the lowest or adhama type means a kumbhaka of sixteen second's duration. Two sittings a day would make a moderate practice, and one sitting every day is sufficient for ordinary purposes. Similarly, the number of rounds: twenty rounds will be enough ordinarily while forty rounds in a sitting would make moderate practice.

One should be very clear about the goal that one wants to reach and decide whether the ordinary, moderate or intense practice is to be followed. Confusion regarding this may be dangerous.

Incessant abdominal breathing : Kapalabhati

While describing the necessity for breathing we have pointed out that oxygen is indispensable for the process of oxidation through which energy is released. In this process while oxygen is utilised two gases are produced: carbon dioxide and water vapour. It is essential to remove these gases out of the body. They are collected by the blood from all over the tissues of the body where oxidation is going on, brought to the lungs, and exchanged there for oxygen from the inhaled air. After this exchange they are eliminated in the following exhalation. When one holds the breath for some time as in kumbhaka this process of elimination of carbon dioxide and water vapour stops for a while. Accumulation of carbon dioxide in the blood beyond a certain limit is dangerous, because it acts as poison and may kill living tissues. To counteract the accumulation of carbon dioxide in the blood there is a technique in yoga which helps to eliminate it faster, so that the composition of the blood becomes normal again. It is called Kapalabhati. Kapala means the skull, and kapalabhati means the technique which makes the skull bright or shining.

The technique of kapalabhati is as follows: Sitting in a posture suitable for pranayama, the student relaxes the wall of the abdomen, contracts the anus, and exhales rapidly and abruptly with some force with a sudden contraction of the abdominal wall just below the navel. By suddenly pulling the abdominal wall towards the back in this manner pressure is exerted inside the abdominal cavity which makes the diaphragm to rise slightly, make an impact on the lungs, and cause a forced exhalation. The abdominal wall is then relaxed again so that the diaphragm comes down, causing vacuum inside the throacic cavity. This vacuum is filled by air entering into the lungs. Then the abdominal wall is immediately contracted again, bringing about another forced exhalation which is followed by inhalation

due to the relaxation of the wall of the abdomen. It is important to note that in this process inhalation is a passive act but
not so exhalation. This is the exact opposite of what happens
in normal breathing where inhalation requires application of
force for contracting the muscles of the chest and exhalation
happens without applying any force, but due to the elastic recoil
of the lungs.

One goes on repeating the process of forced exhalations
twenty, thirty or forty times. When one gets tired the process
may become difficult and the rhythm may be lost. Here one
should stop. All these exhalations done repeatedly in this way
constitute one round. The following points should be noted:

1. Each exhalation should be sudden, not prolonged.
2. While inhaling there should be no effort to suck the air
   in.
3. There should be a fixed rhythm in the process.
4. The chest muscles should not be used.
5. Exhalations and inhalations are to be brought about
   mainly by the movements of the abdominal wall.

Kapalabhati is thus an exercise in rapid abdominal breathing. One may do two exhalations per second. The flow of air
should not be obstructed by contraction of the throat or nose.
But there is slight friction of the air as it comes out and due to
this a low sound is produced. Contraction of the abdominal
wall should be moderate and not vigorous, although it is sudden.
Most of the students can do kapalabhati well on the first day.
But a few find it very difficult to synchronise the movement of
the abdomen with exhalation and inhalation. They contract the
abdominal wall while inhaling. This should be carefully avoided.
On the first day one should do as many exhalations as could be
comfortably and rhythmically performed in a non-stop process.
Then after resting for half a minute another round may be done
and then a third round after half a minute's rest again. The
number of exhalations per round may be increased slowly by
five to ten per week until one can comfortably do each round
for one minute making one hundred twenty exhalations in that
time. This may take about two months from the start.

Normally we inhale and exhale about 500 ml. of air every
time, amounting to a lung ventilation of seven litres of air per
minute. In kapalabhati breathing is slightly deeper so that the

quantity of air respired each time is nearly 600 ml. and there are 120 such respirations per minute. Thus the lung ventilation per minute in kapalabhati increases to 70 litres or more, i.e., it is increased ten times. This helps rapid elimination of carbon dioxide from the blood. Because of this it is observed that after a round of kapalabhati one can hold the breath more easily. In an experiment recently conducted by the present author in this regard (see "Effect of Kapalabhati on Retention of Breath: An Experimental Study" by K.S. Joshi, published in the journal *Yoga Awareness*, February 1981, p. 1-4) it was found that kapalabhati increases the extent of retention of breath significantly in the kumbhakas following a round of kapalabhati and that this increase is the highest in case of the immediately following retention.

Thus it is advisable to do three rounds of kapalabhati in the beginning of a session of pranayama. There is another way in which it may be used while doing pranayama. If one is doing twenty rounds of kumbhaka in a sitting then one round of kapalabhati may be done in the beginning, the second one after six kumbhakas and the third one after six more kumbhakas. This is observed to be of great help for making the kumbhakas comfortable throughout a sitting. Sometimes it is observed that in a sitting the initial kumbhakas are quite comfortable, but toward the end of the sitting there is some uneasiness. One way of overcoming this difficulty is to reduce the duration of each kumbhaka. But perhaps a better way would be to introduce a round of sixty strokes of kapalabhati after six or eight kumbhakas. Here kapalabhati may be said to act like a safety valve for the elimination of accumulated carbon dioxide, which is one main cause of uneasiness during the practice of kumbhaka.

There is an important variety of pranayama in which a round of kapalabhati is introduced before each round of pranayama. That is called Bhastrika pranayama. *Bhastra* means a bellows. This variety of pranayama gets its name from the fact that in every round of it the abdomen is moved like the bellows. Some students and even some teachers of pranayama who are not properly trained are confused between this and kapalabhati and use the word bhastrika for kapalabhati. That may sound reasonable because in kapalabhati also one moves the belly like the bellows. But technically it is wrong, because both bhastrika and kapalabhati are technical terms having fixed or defined meanings, and unless we change the definitions themselves the words should not be used interchangeably.

Kapalabhati is traditionally regarded as one of the cleansing techniques of yoga. There are six main techniques for cleansing different parts of the body. We have already discussed one of these earlier, namely, neti. Kapalabhati may be said to have great significance as a cleansing technique because it cleanses the whole body by removing carbon dioxide which is a poisonous impurity produced continuously in the body. The fact of making the skull or the brain shining is perhaps associated with the impact made by the forcefully outgoing air in each exhalation on the sinuses of the skull and the olfactory mucous membrane. But the exact mechanism involved has not yet been studied.

Holding the breath out

As mentioned earlier there are two ways of doing kumbhaka. We have so far discussed only the more common way, that of holding the breath inside. Holding the breath out, although much less common, is also quite useful from the therapeutic point of view.

It is sometimes recommended by some teachers of pranayama that the two types of kumbhaka are to be practised together in the same round, that is, one should do puraka, inner kumbhaka, rechaka, and then outer kumbhaka in one round, counting the number of such rounds in a sitting. This is not mentioned in any of the major texts of pranayama. Such a practice would be extremely strenuous. So it is better to practice the inner and outer types of kumbhaka separately.

For practising outer kumbhaka it is not necessary to have any proportional time for puraka and rechaka. Kapalabhati can very well be combined with each round. A convenient procedure would be as follows:

Assuming a convenient posture make a round of sixty strokes of kapalabhati. Make the last exhalation as complete as possible, contracting the anus and the abdominal wall. Close both the nostrils, apply the Jalandhara bandha and hold the

breath out for ten, fifteen, twenty or more seconds, depending
on how long it can be held comfortably. Then give up the
bandhas and have a few normal respirations. Then repeat the
whole procedure for a second round. Four such rounds are
enough in the beginning. The number may be slowly increased
to ten in a period of about four weeks.

After finishing the required number of rounds of outer
kumbhaka one may continue the sitting for the practice of inner
kumbhaka after taking a few normal breaths. Thus instead of
introducing outer kumbhaka in each round of inner kumbhaka
as advocated by some teachers it is far more convenient and
useful to combine the two in the above manner. It is always
advisable to go through a few strokes of kapalabhati before
every round of outer kumbhaka.

Outer kumbhaka is a very good respiratory exercise. When
combined with the practice of inner kumbhaka it greatly
enhances the therapeutic value of the latter. It is not to be used
as a substitute to inner kumbhaka. That is why we do not find
any emphasis on it in the traditional texts. The procedure given
above is also not taken from any text. But the present writer
has found it very convenient to combine outer and inner
kumbhakas, and a very practical and useful way of combining
them is described here.

We have so far described all the aspects of how one should
actually begin the practice of pranayama. When one is established in the practice for some months, it is possible to try the
different varieties of pranayama. We shall describe these varieties in the chapter that follows immediately.

5

Varieties of Pranayama

We have referred to the varieties of pranayama earlier. Now we shall describe them in detail. How many varieties of pranayama are there? How do they differ from each other? Should a student practise them all? Which is the most useful among them? Are there any special advantages associated with particular varieties? These are some of the questions which arise when one thinks about the varieties.

As we have noted earlier these different varieties involve only one form of kumbhaka, i.e., the inner kumbhaka. So far as the kumbhaka is concerned the varieties do not show any difference. Yet in some yoga texts they are called varieties of kumbhaka instead of calling them varieties of pranayama. That is because kumbhaka is traditionally considered to be the most important component of pranayama. That is true from the point of view of an advanced student. But it has not much significance for a beginner who may even skip over the kumbhaka altogether, and still derive enough benefits for the fitness of body and mind.

The varieties differ with regard to puraka and rechaka. Either of them may be done through both the nostrils or only through the left or right one. Since kumbhaka is the most effective part of pranayama, this difference of the use of nostrils while inhaling and exhaling should not really matter much because the technique of kumbhaka is the same in all the varieties. But the ancient texts do speak of special features of different varieties. These need not be studied extensively for deciding their relative merits. But so far no such comparative studies have been made.

The principal varieties of pranayama or kumbhaka are only two, namely *sahita* and *kevala*. Sahita means accompanied by. In this variety kumbhaka is accompanied by puraka and rechaka. This variety can be sub-divided into two, namely, inner kumbhaka and outer kumbhaka. Kevala means alone. This kumbhaka is not related to or associated with puraka or rechaka. How does one practise it, if it is irrespective of them, one may ask. The right answer to this question is that it is not a thing to be practised at all. It just happens. It cannot be brought about. We can bring about puraka, kumbhaka, or rechaka but not kevala kumbhaka. Kevala kumbhaka signifies a state in which breathing just stops without any effort. It is a state of complete stillness of the mind and breath. It is a basic presupposition of Hathayoga that the movement of the mind and breath is interdependent. When one is moving the other moves and when one becomes still the other is completely silent, too. Thus kevala kumbhaka signifies a state of *sahaja samadhi*. Just as this state is not the result of any conscious effort, kevala kumbhaka is also not the product of any practice. It has no varieties or grades and no measurement in terms of space, time, or number of repetitions. These qualifications apply only to sahita kumbhaka.

So the varieties which we shall describe now are all varieties of sahita kumbhaka. It is not at all necessary for a student to learn or practise all the varieties of pranayama. A teacher should, however, know them.

1. Anuloma-viloma

Viloma means produced in the reverse order. This variety gets it a name from the fact that the order of using the nostrils for inhalation and exhalation is reversed every time. In each round one does puraka through the left nostril followed by kumbhaka and rechaka through the right nostril, and then reverses the order to do puraka through the right nostril, then kumbhaka and then rechaka through the left nostril. Thus one round of Anuloma-viloma pranayama includes two each of the three components. In all other varieties each round is made by only one each of the three components. A round consists of all the set of procedure that is repeated again and again.

It is not necessary to repeat the details of procedure, e.g., that one should be uniform, that kumbhaka should always be

accompanied by the three bandhas, and so on. We have already
described these points in detail. They are to be followed in all
the varieties. But there is one important point which we have
not discussed earlier. It also applies equally to all the varieties.
The question is: what should one think or do mentally while
doing pranayama?

Pranayama is a process of silencing the breath resulting in
silencing the mind. Even a few rounds of pranayama of moderate measure properly practised can give the student an experience of peace of mind. To promote this experience and to
get the benefit of the effect of pranayama on the mind the
student should remember some facts about the working of the
mind.

One very conspicuous characteristic of the human mind is
that it always wanders from thought to thought, knowing no rest
at any time except in sleep. Much of this is simply a wasteful
activity which, if minimised, could help the mind to function in
a far better and useful way. For that one must learn to forget
oneself at times, giving up all thoughts about the self and its
relations with the external world as well as the inner world
made by desires, beliefs, emotions and passions. This can be
easily done while doing pranayama. At the start one should
remember that one will not entertain any thought about oneself
or the world during the sitting of pranayama. But the mind cannot remain vacant. It must have something to attend to, to be
attached with or to ponder upon. This something may be pro-
vided by a mantra. In the absence of a mantra the mind may be
attached to the flow of air during puraka and rechaka. During
kumbhaka the mind should also be motionless, not remembering any past incident, not thinking about the future, not utter-
ing any word or visualizing any image. With a little practice
one can start enjoying such a silent, detached state of mind
giving rest to it. It is a state of deep absorption in which
the tensions and conflicts which always disturb the mind are
not working. One should attain such a peaceful state of mind
while doing pranayama of any variety.

Anuloma-viloma pranayama is also called Nadishodhaka
pranayama. Nadi means a channel. Shodhaka means that which
purifies. This variety is called the purifier of the nadis especially
because it helps to clear both the nostrils which are used alter-

natively for inhalation and exhalation. Actually every variety of
pranayama cleanses the nadis, and even kapalabhati which is
not counted traditionally as a variety of pranayama is very useful for that purpose. The word nadi does not mean the
nostrils alone. In yoga it has also another meaning which we
shall explain later.

2. Ujjayi

In this variety both the nostrils are used for puraka and the
left one for rechaka. The sound represented by the letters 'hm'
is to be produced during them, by a partial closure of the
glottis. This sound is a peculiarity of this variety and its name
is derived from this fact. It is also called 'Ujjapi' at some places.
In the *Hathayoga-pradipika* (II. 52) it is said that this variety
of pranayama may be practised even while standing or walking.
Obviously kumbhaka should not be done in that condition. It
is doubtful if there is any advantage to be gained by practising
Ujjayi while standing or walking. It would, indeed, be cumbersome to do such a thing.

3. Suryabhedana

Surya means the sun. Surya-nadi is the right nostril. In this
variety of pranayama the right nostril is used for puraka and
the left one for rechaka. In each round this same procedure is
to be repeated. This may be called a viloma type of pranayama.
It is supposed that in our body the sun is situated near the navel
and the moon in the skull above the hard palate. The moon
has a cooling effect and the sun a heating effect. Perhaps the
concept of the sun has been derived from the fact that the food
we eat is digested in the part of the body near the navel. Digestion is supposed to be brought about by heat and the sun is the
source of that heat. The air taken in through the right nostril is
supposed to make an impact on other forms of vital air in the
body. Due to this impact they are collected near the root of the
navel. This is supposed to have a great significance in the arousal of the kundalini. It has not been possible yet to explain all
these ideas from our knowledge of modern physiology.

4. Bhastrika

This variety of pranayama is different from all other varieties in so far as it includes a few strokes of kapalabhati in the beginning of every round. This may be done in various ways as explained in the *Hathayoga-pradipika* (commentary on II. 64). The text itself has mentioned only one of these ways (II. 62-64) according to which the student should first sit in the Padmasana posture and go through a round of rapid exhalations and inhalations, moving the belly like the bellows of a blacksmith. After the last exhalation of this round (of kapalabhati) one should take a deep breath through the right nostril. After this puraka the breath is to be held inside, closing both the nostrils and applying the bandhas. The following rechaka should be done through the left nostril.

This variety of pranayama is recommended for the purpose of arousing the kundalini quickly. We may say that this variety of Bhastrika pranayama is just a combination of Suryabhedana and Kapalabhati.

In the commentary of *Hathayoga-pradipika* some more ways in which Bhastrika pranayama can be practised are described. They are as follows:

1. In the first round the Kapalabhati part is done through the right nostril, followed by puraka through the right nostril, kumbhaka and rechaka through the left nostril. In the second round the Kapalabhati part is done through the left nostril, then puraka through it, followed by kumbhaka and then the right nostril is used for the following rechaka. Then the order is reversed for the third round and again changed for the fourth round, and so on. Thus this variety amounts to Kapalabhati with Anuloma-viloma pranayama.

2. Instead of using only one nostril for Kapalabhati at a time both the nostrils are alternately used, one for inhalation and the other for exhalation. Thus in the first round the right nostril is used for puraka and the left for rechaka of the Kapalabhati part. Then a deep puraka is done through the right nostril to be followed by kumbhaka and then a deep rechaka through the left nostril. Then in the second round the whole order is reversed, i.e., for Kapalabhati the left nostril is used for puraka and the right for rechaka, then the deep puraka and rechaka

are also done through the left and the right nostrils respectively, kumbhaka being done between the two.

Bhastrika may thus be called the most elaborate variety of pranayama.

The four varieties which we have described so far are more common among the varieties of pranayama mentioned in traditional texts. There are four more varieties which are less common. In two of them puraka is done not through the nose but through the mouth. This is said to produce a cooling effect in the body. They differ from each other only so far as the puraka part is concerned. These two varieties are Shitali and Sitkari. Let us describe their technique in some detail.

5. Shitali

Shitala means pleasantly cold. This variety, as mentioned above, has a cooling effect. Hence its name. Its technique is as follows:

Sitting in a suitable posture, the tongue is drawn out of the mouth and its sides are turned upward to form a channel. During puraka the air is slowly sucked in through this channel. After the puraka the tongue is taken in, the mouth is closed. kumbhaka is done along with the bandhas, and then rechaka is done through both the nostrils. About ten to twenty such rounds may be gone through in a sitting. One enjoys doing Shitali pranayama especially in the summer. It is not to be practised in the cold season. Sucking the air over the wet surface of the tongue produces a cooling effect.

About the effects of Shitali pranayama it is said in the *Hathayoga-pradipika* (II. 57) that by its practice one can overcome diseases of the spleen (and perhaps liver) and also have a control on hunger and thirst. Even poisons like snake venom may be destroyed. These claims are definitely worth investigating on the basis of clinical tests.

6. Sitkari

Sitkara is a sound made by drawing in the breath. This variety of pranayama gets its name from this sound which is produced while doing puraka. The puraka is done through the mouth. For this the mouth is slightly opened, the tongue is slightly pressed against the upper jaw, its tip touching the back side of the upper front teeth. The air is sucked in along the surface of the tongue through the gap between the two jaws. Friction of the air with the moist surface of the tongue gives rise to the sound called sitkara. After the puraka is completed the mouth is shut, kumbhaka is done as in all other cases of pranayama, and then rechaka is done through both the nostrils.

Some people call this Shitakari, *sheeta* meaning cold. But that is a mistake, although it is true that this variety of pranayama can also have a cooling effect like Shitali pranayama. The benefits of this variety as mentioned in traditional texts are: control upon hunger and thirst, overcoming laziness, and a vigorous, healthy, attractive personality like Kamadeva, the god of love.

It may be recommended that when a student gets established in the practice of pranayama he may try the various varieties on a moderate scale. For instance, in winter Suryabhedana may be practised for having the heat effects of the sun, while in summer the cooling varieties may be practised with advantage.

There are two more varieties which are not very commonly practised by students. Their description in different texts varies, so it is difficult to say how exactly they are to be practised. These varieties are: Bhramari and Moorchha. We shall describe them according to two different texts in each case.

7. Bhramari

Bhramara means the bumble bee. Its humming sound is imitated in this variety of pranayama. This sound is produced by the friction of the air with the thin edge of the soft palate which hangs like an arch in the posterior part of the mouth. When one snores while sleeping this sound is produced without one's knowledge because of the vibrations of the edge of the soft palate. But snoring the sound is abrupt and uneven. In Bhramari the sound is produced by systematic smooth movements. It is more pronounced during inhalation than in exhalation. Both the nostrils are to be used in puraka and rechaka. It is more difficult to produce the sound during puraka. It is of a higher pitch. Hence it is said that during puraka the sound is

like that of a male bee and in rechaka it is like a female bee, i.e.,
of a lower pitch. This is according to the *Hathayoga-pradipika*
(II. 67).

In the othe text called *Gheranda Samhita* (V. 77) an altogether different description is found. According to it a student is
advised to practise Bhramari pranayama at midnight when the
atmosphere is completely calm due to all sounds and noise of
creatures being silent. One is asked to cover the ears with the
hands and practise puraka and kumbhaka. Then the student
starts hearing various subtle sounds after a continued practice.
That is Bhramari.

There are two drawbacks in this description. First, it is not
explained whether puraka and rechaka are to be practised in
any particular manner, and if so, in what particular manner.
This makes the description very vague. Secondly, the hearing of
subtle sounds which happens after the arousal of kundalini does
not call for any particular variety of pranayama. It is called
nadanusandhana which is the highest part among the four parts
into which Hathayoga is divided. Perhaps what *Gheranda
Samhita* calls Bhramari is just the hearing of sounds in nadanusandhana, in which one may hear the sound of a bee among
other sounds. But that cannot be called a variety of pranayama
itself. It is in fact an effect of a prolonged practice of pranayama.
So for practical purposes the description in the *Hathayoga-pradipika* seems more useful. The *Gheranda Samhita* speaks of
Bhramari in the higher sense. There is nothing wrong in it. But
it is meant for the adept. A beginner cannot practise it that
way.

Of course Bhramari is not a variety of pranayama for the
beginner. But when an established student starts practising
there is an initial difficulty about producing the correct sound
during puraka. To make the edge of the soft palate vibrate to
produce a low uniform sound is found difficult. To overcome
this difficulty one may in the beginning do the puraka through
one nostril only, instead of using both the nostrils. This way
the sound can be produced with more ease and smoothness.
When the sound starts coming properly after some practise,
one can start using both the nostrils for puraka.

Now about the effects of Bhramari pranayama. When one
is able to get the right type of sound during puraka and

rechaka, one starts enjoying it increasingly day by day. It is very absorbing, and has a very soothing effect on the mind. The mind is to be applied to the hearing of this sound, and thus it becomes very peaceful and silent. To some extent this is achieved even in Ujjayi by hearing the sound produced by closing the glottis partially. But the sound produced in Bhramari is more absorbing and soothing. The sound vibrations make an impact on the brain, and their immediate effect is peace and joy, which are things of greatest value in human life.

8. Moorchha

Moorchha means fainting. This variety of pranayama is so named from the fact that by practising it one goes into a state of stupor. This variety is obviously not for the beginner at all. One is asked to apply the Jalandhara bandha not only during the state of kumbhaka as in all other varieties, but also during the following rechaka. This is a speciality of this variety. There is no special recommendation as to how puraka and rechaka are to be done. So it seems that one is expected to use both the nostrils for them. What happens when the Jalandhara bandha is continued during rechaka? A possible explanation would be that pressure is exerted on the carotid sinus and carotid body located on the carotid artery which supplies blood to the head. There are pressure receptors situated in the carotid sinus which when stimulated by exertion of pressure on these parts bring about a lowering of blood pressure and reflex control of respiration. This may lead to the state of stupor in the long run. Such a state coming about by a long practice of Moorchha pranayama is said to be highly pleasurable and enjoyable. This shows how there is an intimate relation between breath control and mind control.

The above description of this variety is according to the *Hathayoga-pradipika* (II. 69). In the *Gheranda Samhita* (V. 83) a different description is found. It is said that one should do kumbhaka comfortably and apply the mind to the point between the eye brows, called *bhroo madhya* and detach it from all other thoughts. This gives rise to the state of stupor. In that state the mind unites with the soul, and that creates a feeling of joy. Thus according to this text Moorchha pranayama differs from other varieties only in respect of concentrating mentally between the eyebrows. This means that any variety of pranayama can be converted into the state of stupor when practised for sufficiently long time with intensity.

What if we use both the techniques mentioned in the two texts for producing the state of stupor and great joy, one may ask. It may be natural to expect that a two-pronged attack would be more effective. And it seems an important conclusion to draw that whichever variety of pranayama one may be practising, it is possible to have the state of joyful Moorchha through persistant effort with either or both of the modifications during kumbhaka mentioned above.

An interesting question arises here. Can we combine the different varieties of pranayama in various ways instead of practising them strictly according to the procedures mentioned in the texts and thereby get more benefit? For one thing such combinations are not mentioned in traditional writings, and then there may be innumerable combinations possible. We have ourselves recommended for the beginner what may be called a combination of Anuloma-viloma, Bhastrika, and Ujjayi. Such a combination is highly useful not only for the beginner but also for an advanced and even a much advanced student of pranayama. Like this some other combinations may also be tried by enthusiastic and imaginative but cautious students.

Before we end this chapter on the varieties of pranayama there is one more variety mentioned in one of the important texts but not in any other. It may be a debatable point whether this can be given the status of an independent variety or just a specialised technique associated with pranayama. Let us see what the text (*Hathayoga-pradipika* II. 69) has to say about it.

9. Plavini

Plu means to swim or float. *Plava* means floating. *Plavini* is that which makes one float. This variety is described in the text in the following words:

"The *udara* is profusely filled with air taken inside the body. Thereby one can effortlessly float even in deep water like a lotus leaf."

The word Udara means the belly. It is also used to indicate any cavity, including the thoracic cavity. The commentator
of the text has not made it clear as to what meaning of the
word the author has in mind here. Some people seem to believe
that filling the udara with air here means filling the belly by gulping in air. Of course this can be done with a little training. All
of us unknowingly gulp in some air while eating. It comes out
with a peculiar sound in belching. One can learn the technique
of eating air by filling the mouth with air, then closing it,
making the cheeks tight, pressing the lips against each other,
and gulping the air just as we gulp water or food. For Plavini,
the stomach is to be filled with air in this way to a considerable
extent. Then one can just float on the surface of water without
moving the limbs. One should lie on the back and keep the
hands behind the head. This helps to balance the body more
comfortably.

But should one practise pranayama while the stomach is
filled with air? Just as one should never do pranayama soon
after taking food it is not advisable also to do it on a stomach
full of air, because that would interfere with free movement
of the diaphragm and abdominal muscles. There would be an
undue pressure on the stomach wall and the abdominal
viscera. That would be like carrying an unnecessary load while
climbing up and down. Moreover, with the stomach filled with
air one would automatically float on water. So actually there is
no pranayama involved in floating like this. Strictly speaking,
therefore, Plavini is not a variety of pranayama as such.

It is possible to raise a doubt about the meaning of the
word udara in the text. Did the author mean the stomach by
the word? Or did he use the word just to mean filling of the
lungs by the word udara? He has actually used the word
udara to mean the lungs while describing the technique of
Bhastrika pranayma. He says, "Puraka should be done
through the right nostril (after the Kapalabhati part) till the
udara is completely filled with air." Nobody will translate the
word 'udara' here to mean the stomach. It clearly means the
chest, or rather the lungs. And this is not the only example in
the traditional texts where udara means the chest cavity. So it
is quite likely that the author of the text really meant by the
phrase 'filling the udara with air' nothing else but taking long

breaths and then holding the breath. Understood this way, the verse may become meaningful. Plavini may then mean doing kumbhaka while lying on the back on the surface of water. This can actually be done with some practice. The present writer has taught this technique to many students. Of course one must know swimming well already. If one takes the hands behind the head and keeps the chin away from the chest, bending the neck backward as one does in Matsyasana, then one can float in a horizontal position without effort. This is helped by doing kumbhaka as air is much lighter than water. This kumbhaka, which in fact is like any other example of kumbhaka of the inner type, may be called plavini because it helps one to float.

To sum up so far: we have pointed out in this chapter that there are only two principal varieties of pranayama, namely, sahita and kevala. Sahita is of two types, called *bahya* and *abhyantara*. We have described nine varieties of the latter.

This completes our discussion of the question: How is pranayama to be practised, and in how many ways can the practice be followed. The next question that we shall discuss would be: What are the effects of pranayama on the body. For discussing those effects we must first explain the process of breathing in detail, so that we can bring out the changes that pranayama gives rise to. To this task let us now turn.

6

Pranayama: A Key to Good Health

What are the advantages one can derive from a regular practice of pranayama? This is the topic we shall discuss in this chapter. It is good for every student of pranayama to have a clear idea of this so as to get the highest benefit from the practice. The main import of this whole book is that pranayama is a key to good health. We have described already how to use the key. How that key works is what we shall discuss now. First we must see what is the importance of health and then what constitutes good health.

Importance of good health

All of us know the proverb "If health is lost, everything is lost." There are many things in our life of which we are hardly ever aware when they are there, but the moment they are gone we become aware of them by feeling their absence. Health is one such thing. When it is there we do not remember it always, although it expresses itself in everything that we do. The importance of the saying "health is wealth" is felt more when health is impaired.

If we watch the behaviour of each one of us in daily life it would be found that everyone is striving for reaching some goal or achieving something. There are nearer and farther goals varying from individual to individual and from time to time. But there is one common goal for all of us, and that is lasting happiness. This may be called the essence of all our activities. Through everything that we do we desire to achieve lasting happiness. What is the principal means that we have for achieving the goal of happiness? Obviously it is our body and mind. Unless this is in a good condition one cannot enjoy happiness even if money, fame, and position exist. So health is of supreme importance.

Importance of health in life can hardly be over-emphasised. To have a healthy body (and mind) is an asset perhaps more important than having good education, good parents, and inheritance of riches. Happiness may be said to be more intimately related to good health than to these outer factors. In the wake of all luxuries if health is lacking then happiness certainly becomes a far cry. Of course, other means must also be there, but without health they have very little meaning.

It is hardly enough simply to know that health has great importance. All of us do know this fact. What is perhaps more important to know is what are the essential conditions to be fulfilled for being a healthy individual.

What constitutes health

Among the factors that influence health we may distinguish between the external factors and the internal ones. Environmental conditions, heredity, pattern of behaviour or way of life, work and rest, food habits, cleanliness, and exercise may be mentioned as some of the external factors that go to decide whether an individual will be healthy or otherwise. We shall leave the discussion of these factors to the next chapter. Here we shall be concerned more with the internal components of health.

If we are asked to imagine a healthy individual and tell what is the most outstanding feature of health, then most of us would come out with the ideas such as a good muscular built, lot of physical power and strength of muscles. But these are not the essential or necessary qualities of a healthy person. These qualities may be essential for warriors, players, or athletes but not for the common man. Perhaps vitality and endurance may be described as essential qualities even for the common man. These are directly related to a healthy condition of the body. So far as the muscles are concerned flexibility may be considered as more important than physical strength. In the present age of mechanical power not many of us are required to exert physically. A century ago when people were required to ride on horseback and carry loads physically, muscle power was more important, but now the situation is changed. But good muscular strength is of course valuable.

It is necessary for health that all the functions going on in the body must be carried on perfectly well. Our body works like an extremely elaborate machine. Even in a simple machine one faulty part means loss of efficient working. This is very true of the human body also. Only when each function in the body goes on properly it can be called a state of health. The main functions in the human body are: intake, digestion and assimilation of food, circulation of blood, secretion of fluids and harmones, respiration, removal of waste materials, conduction of impulses and sensations, and co-ordination of various activities. To this list we must add reproduction and intellection as very important functions. If any of the specialised organs and systems connected with these functions is defective then one is not healthy, however physically strong one may be. Health is a state which is the sum total of all these bodily functions.

Health is not a mere bodily phenomenon alone. It has a psychological aspect as well. Full mental growth is a necessary component of health. In case of animals bodily strength is all that may constitute health. But in case of man a healthy mind is as important or even more important than a healthy body. Mentally backward or underdeveloped persons cannot be said to enjoy full health even if they may be very fit bodily. "Healthy mind in a healthy body" is a saying that is true generally, but not necessarily in each and every case.

Mental health requires two qualities in addition to intellectual ability, namely, mental poise or balance, and sense of values. Our mind is full of attitudes, likes and dislikes, emotions, desires, fears and beliefs. Each one of us also has a set of values involving ideas about wrong and right, good and bad, and the highest goal and the ideal of man. When there is a balance and order among these ideas and tendencies one is apt to be mentally healthy. When a balance or poise is lacking and when some of these go out of hand that results into ill health. When one has improper goals and inadequate sense of values one is definitely lacking in sound mental health.

In sum, health is a state of an individual made by vitality, endurance, flexibility of body and mind, and a kind of balance and order in all the functions of body and mind. Such a state cannot come about by itself. It requires attention and care. In this chapter it shall be our endeavour to show how pranayama can be of great help in this regard, and how pranayama can be used as a key to good health. Before we can discuss how pranayama works as a key it would be necessary to understand thoroughly the process of breathing, how it goes on normally, and how it is modified in pranayama. We shall therefore describe here some physiological facts about breathing which a student of pranayama should know.

Mechanism of breathing

As noted earlier we go on breathing in and out without usually noticing it. For breathing in we have to put in effort for expanding the chest so that the lungs also open up to admit air from the atmosphere which comes in through the nose and the wind pipe to fill the vacuum created by expansion of the lungs. The thoracic cavity in which the lungs are placed, is made by twelve pairs of ribs. They are attached in front to the chest bone and posteriorly to the back bone. By contraction of the external intercostal muscles placed between the ribs, the ribs slightly rotate around the joints with the back bone. The sternum (chest bone) moves upward and forward with the ribs. At the same time the diaphragm which forms the base of the thoracic cavity contracts and moves downward, thus expanding the chest cavity. Thus inspiration takes place. In inspiration the lungs extend passively in response to the decreasing pressure on them due to the expansion of the thoracic cavity. In expiration the abdominal muscles contract, squeezing the abdominal viscera against the liver. At the same time the diaphragm relaxes and it is pushed up, pulling the sternum and the ribs down. This is aided by the elastic recoil of the lungs. The thoracic volume is decreased and the air is forced out of the lungs.

The lungs are not completely filled or emptied in each respiratory cycle in normal quiet breathing. Each time we normally take in and force out about 500 ml. of air. This is called tidal volume. After such a normal exhalation we can draw out a further quantity of one litre of air in forced exhalation. This is called expiratory reserve volume. The lungs are not fully

emptied even at this stage. They still hold about 1200 ml. of air.
This air cannot be forced out of the lungs in spite of all effort.
This is called residual volume. The volume of air that can be
taken in with a maximum inspiration is called inspiratory
capacity. That is about 3500 ml. After such an inspiration the
lungs hold nearly five litres of air, which is called total lung
capacity. The maximum amount of air that a person can draw
out after taking a deep breath is called the vital capacity. It is
an important indicator of health as it gives information about
the strength of the respiratory muscles, the distensibility of the
lungs and the size of the thoracic cage. Under Indian conditions
an average person has a vital capacity of about four litres.
Women have a smaller vital capacity than this. In western
countries the average is much more.

Exchange of gases in the lungs

The atmospheric air entering the lungs contains roughly
79% nitrogen, 20% oxygen, and traces of carbon dioxide. Out
of these only oxygen is of use to the body. In exchange for
it the body gives carbon dioxide and water vapour. The lungs
provide a vast area for this gaseous exchange. The wind pipe
(trachea) divides into two bronchi. Each bronchus enters the
lung on its side and divides itself into several branches called
bronchioles. The bronchioles further divide and sub divide
themselves into fine terminal branches, which in the end fork
into the true respiratory bronchioles which hold the minute air
sacks called alveoli, which have a very thin lining through
which gases can pass. The alveoli are surrounded with extremely
thin walled capillaries through which blood flows. Each
alveolus is an extremely small microscopic structure, but the
number of alveoli in the lungs is enormous. They are all together estimated to provide a surface area of nearly 50 square
metres for an exchange of gases. The amount of blood flowing
through the capillaries in the lungs is about 60 to 80 ml. This
allows a fairly quick exchange of gases inside the lungs,
because a small quantity of blood is spread over a large surface
area.

All the air we inhale in each respiration does not reach the
alveoli. Some of it remains in the nose, trachea and bronchi,

and contains part of exhaled air which is inhaled again in the following respiration. This is known as the dead space. It is about 150 ml., so that in each respiration only 350 ml. of fresh air reaches the alveoli. Thus in quiet breathing about five litres of fresh air enters the lungs every minute. This is called the minute volume.

Over the surface of the alveoli gaseous exchange takes place between the air contained in the alveoli and the blood circulating through the capillaries surrounding them. This is possible because of two things: first, the membranes of the alveoli and the capillaries are so thin that gases can diffuse through them freely, and second, there is difference in the pressures exerted by the gases on the two sides. In a mixture of gases each gas exerts its pressure proportional to its concentration in the mixture. Air is a mixture of gases. In the alveolar air the partial pressure of oxygen, also called oxygen tension, is 105 mm. of mercury, while that in the blood in the capillaries is 40 mm. Hg. The partial pressure of carbon dioxide in the alveolar air is 40 mm. Hg., while that of the blood is 45 mm. Hg., or more. It is observed that when two gases or mixtures of gases are separated by a semi-permeable membrane, molecules of gas move from the side of higher tension to the side of lower tension. This is known as the law of diffusion. Thus in case of the alveoli and capillaries of the lungs, oxygen moves from the air to the blood and carbon dioxide and water vapour diffuse from the blood to the alveolar air. The oxygen is quickly absorbed by the hemoglobin in the blood.

The rate of diffusion of gases depends upon the tension gradient or the difference between the partial pressures of gas on the two sides of the semi-permeable membrane. With a sharp difference there is rapid diffusion.

Absorption of oxygen and elimination of carbon dioxide and water vapour is the essence of respiration. This process goes on continuously in us as long as we live, without in any way requiring our attention. According to the needs of the body necessary modifications are brought about in the whole process of respiration. These changes are governed by the nervous system.

Nervous control of respiration

We can never forget to breathe because the mechanism controlling breathing is not dependent on our attention. Breathing involves a highly coordinated activity of different sets of muscles such as the muscles of the abdominal wall, the diaphragm, the muscles between the ribs, and also muscles in the neck. Coordination between these muscles is achieved through specialized groups of nerve cells situated in the medulla oblongata of the hind brain, the area of the hind-brain known as the pons and specialized groups of cells in the mid brain. The medulla oblongata is a part of the nervous system situated between the brain and spinal cord. Under normal conditions the respiratory centre in the medulla goes on sending impulses to the muscles of respiration rhythmically to bring about inspiration and expiration alternatingly. This centre is divided into two parts. The ventrally situated part is called the 'inspiratory centre'. It is connected with the diaphragm and the external intercostal muscles through motor nerves and with the walls of the alveoli of the lungs through sensory nerves. When stimulated, this centre causes the muscles to contract, which results in inspiration. The dorsally located part of this respiratory centre is called 'expiratory centre'. It is connected with the abdominal muscles and the internal intercostal muscles. When these muscles contract under impulses from the centre, expiration follows.

In normal quiet breathing the inspiratory centre sends impulses to the muscles of inspiration which are weak in the beginning of inspiration. They grow increasingly stronger as inspiration proceeds so as to overcome resistance offered by the chest muscles and the walls of the alveoli. The stretch receptors in the walls of the alveoli start sending inhibitory impulses to the inspiratory centre when the alveoli get filled with air. When these inhibitory impulses grow strong due to the stretching of the walls of the alveoli, they stop the impulses from the inspiratory centre. At this stage the expiratory centre starts sending its impulses to the muscles to bring about expiration. The muscles of inspiration relax. The alveoli shrink and the inhibitory impulses starting from them fade away. Then the inspiratory centre takes charge again, and the cycle goes on repeating itself.

The amount of carbon dioxide in the blood has a great influence on the respiratory centre. When the concentration of carbon dioxide rises as in exercise or any strenuous work, it stimulates the cells of the respiratory centre, especially the inspiratory centre. This results in an increased rate of respiration, and elimination of the extra amount of carbon dioxide.

The centre in the pons regulates the alternate activity of the inspiratory and expiratory centres in the medulla. It is called the pneumotaxic centre. It is influenced by the chemoreceptors situated in the carotid bodies which are sensitive to decreased oxygen content of blood. We have already referred to the carotid sinus which has presso-receptors which play a role in bringing about a state of stupor through an influence on the pneumotaxic centre.

When one holds the breath, inhibitory impulses from the cortical and subcortical areas of the brain are brought to bear on the respiratory centre, stopping its activity for a short time. This cannot be done indefinitely because when the carbon dioxide concentration of the blood increases beyond a certain limit the respiratory centre overpowers these higher inhibitory impulses and breathing follows in spite of all the efforts to stop it.

Breathing under abnormal conditions

So far we have discussed the process of breathing under normal conditions. Although the life of most of us passes under more or less normal conditions so far as breathing is concerned, abnormalities do sometimes arise due to various reasons, and breathing is modified. Pranayama introduces modifications of breathing. But they are different from modifications introduced by abnormal conditions. Before we go to study the modifications brought about by pranayama it would be to our advantages to see how breathing is modified due to abnormalities of the external and internal environment.

First we shall consider abnormalities of the external environment. These pertain mainly to atmospheric pressure and humidity. At rest our body utilises about 250 ml. of oxygen and gives out 250 ml. of carbon dioxide per minute. At sea level with the atmospheric pressure of 760 mm. Hg., and oxygen concentration of 20% in the air, we should need to breathe only about 1.25 litres of air per minute to fulfil the oxygen requirements of the body. But actually we breathe 6 to 7 litres of air every minute. This is because not all the air we take in reaches the alveoli. We do not absorb all the oxygen contained in the air. Had it been otherwise, i.e., if we could absorb all the oxygen in the inspired air in each breath and if all the air could be driven out every time, filling the lungs with fresh air, then our breathing pattern would have been much different. Because of the dead space we inhale some of the air driven out of the alveoli again in the next inspiration. That air contains only 16% oxygen. So we have to breath in more air.

We can breathe comfortably upto an oxygen content of the air as low as 12%. Below this level it becomes difficult to absorb oxygen into the blood because of a lowering of the tension gradient which slows down the process of diffusion. At high altitudes the atmospheric pressure decreases and the concentration of oxygen in the air goes on reducing as one goes to higher and higher altitudes. The ventilatory rate is increased and one gasps for air. It causes symptoms like nausea, headache and delusions, known as altitude sickness. To overcome the lack of oxygen in the atmosphere at such heights one has to breathe in pure oxygen.

Asphyxiation or acute lack of oxygen causes a failure of the nervous mechanism controlling respiration resulting into convulsive breathing. The inspiratory and expiratory muscles may contract simultaneously.

Excess of carbon dioxide is quite dangerous to life. Normally the atmosphere contains only traces of it (0.03%). Exhaled air contains nearly 4% carbon dioxide. Upto 5% concentration of CO_2 in the atmosphere there is not much difficulty in breathing. Concentrations higher than this give rise to acidosis and a higher concentration of CO_2 in the blood acts as poison. To eliminate extra carbon dioxide from the body the ventilatory rate is increased by stimulation of the respiratory centre. There is also an increase in the amount of blood circulating through the lungs.

Water vapour is a constituent of the atmospheric and alveolar air. In humid atmospheres the amount of water vapour in the air is greatly increased. It lowers the partial pressure of oxygen which necessitates more intake of air in respiration. When the air is abnormally hot and dry it has a destructing effect on the membrane of the respiratory passage. We are not usually aware of the fact that we are breathing out water vapour while exhaling. This fact becomes evident on cool dry mornings when the vapour given out is quickly liquified due to cold and it comes out like a jet especially if drawn out through the mouth.

Abnormalities of the internal environment are usually pro- duced by disorders of the lungs and heart. In pneumothorax air enters between the two-layered covering of the lung (pleural cavity) either by accident or for treatment. This causes the lung to collapse and results in serious respiratory difficulties. In tuberculosis the lung tissue is destroyed, which reduces the respiratory efficiency. In pleurisy there may be inflammation of the pleura and accumulation of fluid in the pleural cavity. This causes great difficulty in breathing. In asthma the smooth muscles in the walls of the bronchioles contract excessively which narrows down the respiratory passage and interferes with breathing. All these abnormalities need very careful attention.

We are now in a position to see how breathing is modified in pranayama and what effects these modifications may bring about on the working of the various systems in the body. After discussing these effects the utility of pranayama as a caretaker of health will become clear.

Effects of pranayamic breathing

Among the various activities going on in our body some are fully under our control while others are not. Those activiti- es which are brought about by voluntary muscles can be done at our will. For instance, we can raise a hand and bring it down whenever we like. Movements of the limbs, mouth, eyelids, neck, back, and so on can be done as and when we wish. But this is not the case with all activities. Those activities which are governed by the automatic nervous system cannot be modified by us. Working of the heart, circulation of blood, secretion of digestive juices and hormones, digestion and assimilation of food, are some of the activities which are not under our control. Modifications in these activities come about not by our will but by the homeostatic balance systems in the body.

Respiration is an activity which falls midway between these two types. It is usually modified automatically according to requirements of the body, and this happens without awareness. To some extent we can also modify it voluntarily. If we so desire, we can breathe rapidly, or slowly, deeply or superficially, and we can even stop breathing for a short time. This is possible, first, because there are respiratory centres which govern the activity of respiration, and secondly because we can inhibit their activity by impulses from the brain. That is why pranayama is possible at all.

For bringing out the effects of pranayamic breathing we must consider what things we specially do in pranayama and what their effects are. The special features of pranayama are: 1. An erect sitting posture, 2. Relaxation of the body and mind, 3. Complete filling and emptying of the lungs, 4. Changes in lung ventilation, 5. Pressure changes in the thoracic and abdominal cavities, 6. Exercise of the muscles of respiration, and 7. Activation of hitherto silent areas of the nervous system. We have already made references to these special features in passing in the earlier chapters. Here we shall consider them one by one in detail.

ERECT SITTING POSTURE

While one sits with the back, neck and head erect there is a slight upward stretch exercised along the back and the abdominal wall. Those of us who have to do a sitting job, e.g., tailors, typists, clerks, and who usually keep the body in a slightly bending forward position for a long time everyday, find that after some time their digestive system becomes weak and disorders of the gastrointestinal tract start developing, especially if they are not doing any regular exercise. This tendency can be checked by developing a habit of sitting straight. By the stretch on the abdominal muscles their tone is improved. Sagging of the belly can be stopped. The slight pressure on the abdominal

viscera in the straight sitting position helps to remove congestion of blood and improve the function of all the organs in the
abdominal cavity. This has a very beneficial effect on the general
health of an individual.

Keeping the back straight is very useful for removing
postural defects. Pain in the back, which is a common complaint
of middle aged persons can be removed by the straight sitting
posture. The pull on the spine is a very useful characteristic of
the meditative postures of pranayama. It has great significance
for an arousal of the Kundalini. For the common man it is of
great use for removing undue pressure due to faulty posture on
parts of the vertebral column which may result in severe conditions like spondylitis.

RELAXATION OF THE BODY AND MIND

While practising pranayama the whole body is held in a
relaxed condition. Relaxation is a very useful art. It is a quality
of the muscles and of the mind. A new born child relaxes completely when its bodily needs are fulfilled. Animals are also
found to be completely relaxing when there is no work and the
belly is full. All of us are born with the capacity to relax but
when we grow this capacity is lost because we forget the art of
'letting go' which is the essence of relaxation. Tension is the
opposite of relaxation. Where there is tension there is no relaxation, and vice versa. In daily life we need both tension and
relaxation. Both have a role to play. Without tension there
would be no movement of a muscle. Each muscle is a bundle of
minute fibres of tissue which has two qualities, namely, exten-
sibility and contractibility. When a muscle receives impulses
from a motor nerve it responds to the impulse by shortening its
length, i.e., by contracting. Or it may be stretched, which is a
state of tension. When an impulse is withdrawn the muscle
assumes its normal resting length and there is no tension. This
is the state of relaxation. When all the fibres constituting a
muscle are relaxing it may be called deep relaxation. But usually
some fibres remain under tension, giving rise to only partial
relaxation of the muscle.

Unless there is some tension in the mind we would not
think anything. A continuous relaxed state of the muscle or of

the mind would mean inaction. Such a thing is not desirable because it would adversely influence our daily activities which are most essential.

It is necessary that there is a balance between tension and relaxation. Neither of the two should get out of hand. Tension is necessary for activity, while relaxation is essential for rest. Excess of any one of the two is undesirable. It is observed that whenever there is tension in the mind due to any cause such as fear, frustration of desire, and excitement, that causes tightening of the muscles in different parts of the body. On the other hand, if the muscles are held relaxed then tension from the mind also vanishes. That is why relaxation helps to overcome tensions in the mind.

In pranayama all the muscles are relaxed, contracting only the respiratory muscles in the acts of puraka and rechaka. This helps to give the body and mind complete rest and eliminate tensions from the mind. This has a great influence on the physiological functions of the body. In a recent study made by the present writer on the substitutes to Mahesh Yogi's transcendental meditation (published in the *Yoga Mimamsa* Journal, Vol. XVIII, 1976, pp. 63-67) it was found that effects similar to those claimed for TM of Mahesh Yogi were found in case of participants in the experiment who practised guided relaxation, external kumbhaka, Anuloma-viloma pranayama, and meditation of the Pranava japa type. It was observed that by practising any one of these techniques for twenty to thirty minutes, pulse rate, blood pressure and respirations per minute were reduced, skin resistance was increased (indicating a peaceful state of mind), and the brain activity in terms of frequency and amplitude of the brain waves was considerably silenced.

This influence of pranayama on slowing down the physiological functions can be made use of in overcoming many types of psychosomatic illness. The physiological effects of relaxation may be summarised in the following manner. Relaxation of muscles means withdrawal of impulses to them and lowering of expenditure of energy. The latter causes the heart to pump the blood more slowly and gives it rest by lowering its work load. The former makes the brain silent.

FILLING AND EMPTYING OF THE LUNGS

Normal quiet breathing is very shallow as compared to pranayamic breathing. In successive deep breaths one can inhale and exhale more than four litres of air each time. But in normal breathing only one eighth of this capacity is used. In pranayama one breathes to one's full capacity every time, filling and emptying the lungs to the maximum possible extent. All the alveoli are stretched fully in puraka and shrink fully in rechaka. This promotes blood circulation in all the parts of the lungs and helps diffusion of gases on a larger scale. Normally the upper portions of the lungs near the apex do not expand and contract appreciably in shallow breaths. In pranayama they are also filled and emptied. It is observed that any part of our body which remains inactive for a long time loses its tone and efficiency, its blood circulation becomes sluggish, there may be congestion of blood, and accumulation of waste materials. This makes the part concerned more prone to infection and decay. Lung affections like tuberculosis are thus more commonly observed in the upper parts which are comparatively inactive. Pranayama can surely be said to remove this possibility, of course, it is neither necessary nor desirable to fill the lungs completely in each breath all the twenty four hours of the day. That would certainly be very hazardous. But a few rounds of pranayama each day are certainly very useful for maintaining the respiratory system in a healthy condition.

INFLUENCE ON VENTILATORY RATE

Since the chief aim of respiration is to supply enough quantities of oxygen in the alveolar air for diffusion into the blood in the lung capillaries, any technique that promotes this must be considered very good for health. It is believed, by and large, that pranayama makes us absorb more oxygen or prana and thus improves vital health. Let us see how far this belief is true.

Absorption of oxygen depends on two factors, namely, ventilatory rate and the relative oxygen tension inside the alveoli and capillaries. Ventilatory rate means the quantity of fresh air reaching the alveoli per minute. If this is increased then the absorption of oxygen can increase. The oxygen tension of the alveolar air is 105 mm. Hg., while that of the blood is 40 mm. Hg. Normally the ventilatory rate is 5 litres per minute. In Kapalabhati it increases to 50 to 60 litres per minute. Thus in Kapalabhati more oxygen is absorbed into the blood and carbon dioxide is removed more rapidly. This makes the respiratory centre calm and therefore one can hold the breath comfortably for a longer time immediately following a round of Kapalabhati. But does this happen in pranayama also?

In pranayama not involving retention of breath if one does four rounds of puraka and rechaka in one minute, the ventilatory rate will be about sixteen litres per minute. This will be advantageous for absorption of oxygen and removal of carbon dioxide. If only two rounds are made in a minute, doing puraka for ten seconds and rechaka for twenty seconds, then one would respire eight litres of air per minute But if kumbhaka is practised even for ten seconds in a round, then the minute volume is reduced, and one would not be in an advantageous position so far as oxygen absorption and carbon dioxide elimination is concerned. Introduction of a round of Kapalabhati after four or six rounds of kumbhaka would put the student in an advantageous position again.

Thus, during pranayama itself one may not absorb more oxygen. But pranayama does improve the function of respiration by giving exercise to the muscles of respiration and by its influence on the respiratory centres. Thereby one is apt to respire more efficiently throughout the day. This is one great advantage of pranayama.

PRESSURE CHANGES IN THE THORACIC AND ABDOMINAL CAVITIES

The throacic cavity is made by the rib cage on the sides and the diaphragm at the bottom. The abdominal cavity has the wall of the abdomen in front, the vertebral column on the back and the pelvis at the bottom. Both these cavities expand and contract alternately during respiration due to the movement of the diaphragm and the abdominal muscles. As the cavity expands the pressure inside is reduced, while it is increased as the cavity assumes a smaller size. This pressure works on the organs contained in the two cavities. During inspiration the pressure inside the thoracic cavity is lower than atmospheric pressure. So the lungs are filled with air. At this time the pressure inside the abdominal cavity increases because of the descending diaphragm. During expiration the pressure inside the abdominal cavity is released by the ascent of the diaphragm and that inside the thoracic cavity increases, driving out the air through the respiratory passage. These pressure changes are enhanced highly during pranayama because of taking complete breaths. This has a twofold effect. First, it promotes blood circulation in both the cavities because when the difference in pressure inside the two cavities is greatly increased the blood rushes more rapidly from the high pressure area to the low pressure area. Secondly, due to changing pressures on the internal organs they are squeezed and released alternatively so that a mild exercise is given to the tissues of the organs. Bandhas applied during pranayama play a major role in this, subjecting the heart, the lung tissue, the stomach, intestines, kidneys, liver, pancreas, and the thyroid, parathyroid, and adrenal glands to alternate high and low pressures. All these organs get enough blood supply, and the health and efficiency of all of them is improved. This is one important point in favour of pranayama which makes it a key to good health.

EXERCISE OF THE MUSCLES OF RESPIRATION

In normal respiration particular sets of muscles contract and relax rhythmically to bring about inspiration and expiration. In pranayama these muscles are regulated in their activity with far greater control and the force of contraction on them is sustained for a fairly long time. In puraka the external intercostal muscles, the diaphragm and the muscles of the neck and upper back are contracted, not all of a sudden and for a short time as in the case of a normal inspiration, but slowly, progressively, and for a longer time. Similarly-in rechaka the abdominal muscles and the internal intercostal muscles are contracted. While the inspiratory muscles are contracting the expiratory muscles go on relaxing, and vice versa. Toward the end of puraka and rechaka the abdominal muscles are contracted. During kumbhaka all the contracted muscles are held tight in that position, and in addition to this contractions of muscles involving the bandhas are also brought into play.

A muscle can contract in three different ways. (i) When a muscle shortens in length quickly, bringing about movement of a bone or other part to which it is attached, it is called isotonic contraction. (ii) When a stretched muscle comes back to its normal resting length by a gradual release of tension, it is called eccentric contraction. (iii) In isometric contraction a muscle is held under tension without causing a change in its length. Exercises like running, swimming, sun-prostrations (Surya-namaskara), sit-ups, and so on, involve isotonic contraction. In pranayama the contraction of muscles of respiration is more of an eccentric and isometric type. It involves less energy expenditure. It is far more efficient for developing endurance and flexibility of a muscle as compared to isotonic contraction.

Thus pranayama may be said to ensure a strong and efficient muscle system concerning respiration, which means efficient functioning of the respiratory system. And this influence is not limited to the respiratory system alone, because the abdominal muscles, the diaphragm, and the muscles contracted for the bandhas do help to improve practically every function going on in the body.

ACTIVATION OF HITHERTO SILENT AREAS OF THE BRAIN

Neurologists tell us that out of the over six billion cells in the brain we actually use only a small portion for our activities, both bodily and mental, throughout our life. If all the silent areas of the brain could be brought into action then one could become a superman. But nothing is known scientifically yet about that possibility. Perhaps the masters of pranayama of ancient times had an idea of this. Patanjali, for instance, when he said that pranayama dispels the veil of ignorance which covers the light of knowledge, and it makes the mind fit to be silent in the state of dharana (*Yogasutra*, II. 52, 53.), possibly had in mind this phenomenon of bringing into activity the silent areas of the brain. And although the details of this phenomenon might or might not have been clear in the times of Patanjali, its effects were experienced by the masters of pranayama. There are many such references to the higher effects of pranayama in ancient yoga literature.

We can have some idea of how the effects may be produced if we consider what is happening in the nervous system while doing pranayama. While doing puraka the normal working pattern of the inspiratory centre is modified by impulses from the brain. In rechaka the expiratory centre is receiving impulses from the brain. Stronger impulses than these are associated with the state of kumbhaka. Usually one is not accustomed to bring in these impulses, and the area where they are generated and the pathways along which they flow are silent. When one gets established in the practice of pranayama this area and the pathway becomes quite active. It is very likely that the hypothalamus which is an important relay centre of the brain may be associated with these newly opened pathways. The hypothalamus is connected with a variety of functions, such as integration of autonomic activity, control of emotions, regulation of body temperature, food intake, thirst, endocrine secretions, and sexual behaviour. It is interesting to note that among the effects of pranyama mentioned in the ancient texts we find the following: (i) profuse sweating, (ii) reduction of hunger, thirst, and sleep, (iii) silencing of the mind, (iv) reduction in the production of urine and feaces, and so on. Many of these functions are governed by the hypothalamus.

Of course, for producing the higher effects as mentioned above it is necessary to do pranayama for a long time and in a large measure. But the brain centres and the new pathways of impulses are activated even with a moderate practice of pranayama which is within the reach of the common man. With just a little practice of pranayama one can experience peace of mind, lowering of tensions, a feeling of well-being and a kind of orderliness and discipline in one's behaviour in daily life. Thus pranayama can have an all round improvement in one's personality.

Another higher effect of pranayama to which there are numerous references in ancient texts, is an arousal of the dormant power called Kundalini. Not much is known to modern physiology yet about this mysterious power. So we have to depend upon what is said about it in the texts of yoga and Tantra. It is said that this power is coiled up at the base of the Susumna nadi in the Mooladhara lotus. Due to a prolonged practice of kumbhaka the two vayus, prana and apanao make a joint impact on the kundalini. This impact is made more effective by the bandhas. This awakens the kundalini. It leaves its coiled form, becomes straight, and starts rising up through the lotuses placed inside the Susumna. When it reaches the Anahata lotus at the heart and opens it up, prana follows it there and gets stabilized. This results into hearing of subtle sounds called Anahata-dhvani. One starts hearing sounds resembling those of the sea, clouds, drums, bells, humming of the bee, and in the end one hears sounds of the string instrument (*vina*) and flute. When the sound begins one is advised to apply the mind to the hearing of the sound. It is so absorbing that the mind gets extremely still, giving up all its habit of wandering. Just as a deer is caught up in the net of the hunter or a snake is made motionless by the snake-charmer, the mind loses all its movements and gets absorbed into the sound. The sound goes on becoming subtler with time and becomes silent ultimately. With it the mind reaches a state of complete stillness. This is the state of kevala kumbhaka which makes all further practice of pranayama wholly unnecessary.

After this culmination of the practice of pranayama the kundalini rises higher into the Ajnya chakra which is called the seat of the mind, and ultimately merges itself with the Supreme Lord in the Sahasrara chakra inside the brain. The highest state of mukti-nirvana, or emancipation thus comes into being. We find a very lucid description of all this in the *Yogataravali*, a composition of 27 verses by the great Shankaracharya, and also in the *Shatchakra-nirupana* of Poornananda.

Thus emancipation is what pranayama ultimately leads to. We have just mentioned it here without offering any explanations of the process involved with a view to show that the ancient masters had very high ideals to be reached by pranayama practice, and that the nearer and smaller goals which are useful for all of us are not all that pranayama offers.

We have so far discussed in some detail the effects, both near and far, that a regular practice of pranayama produces.

Now let us see how these various effects make pranayama a key to good health.

Pranayama: a key to good health

We have defined health as a state of an individual which is a sum total of vitality, endurance, flexibility, and balance of the various functions. We shall now see how these pre-requisites of health are all fulfilled by a regular practice of pranayama. First of all, the effect of pranayama on the various functions. The functions which we must consider are: digestion, circulation, respiration, secretion, excretion, reproduction, and co-ordination.

DIGESTION

The digestive system starts with the mouth and extends upto the anus. The whole tract is about thirty feet in length. The items of food are ground to paste in the mouth and are gulped down the pharynx through the oesophagus to the stomach. In the stomach and the part following it called duodenum the food is mixed with digestive juices which break down the carbohydrates, fats, and proteins to simpler substances like glucose, fatty acids, and amino acids respectively. These are then absorbed in the intestines and the waste materials are passed on the large intestine from where they are eliminated in the form of feaces through the anus. The liver and pancreas are very important glands in the abdominal cavity which are intimately associated with digestion. Debility of any part of the digestive system may result in disorders like hyper and hypo acidity, lack of appetite, gases, constipation, and so on.

Pranayama helps to keep the organs of digestion in a fit condition in the following manner:

    (i) By exerting high and low pressure alternating the tone of the organs is improved.

    (ii) Each organ gets enough blood supply whereby nutrients are provided copiously and waste materials are removed efficiently.

(iii) Both the above circumstances help to ensure good appetite, complete digestion and assimilation, and regular evacuation. This has a good effect on all the activities of an individual, because it ensures sufficient supply of energy which is required for any activity.

(iv) The abdominal muscles become strong and the tendency for accumulation of fat on the belly is reduced.

CIRCULATION OF BLOOD

Nutrients required by any part of the body are collected by the blood from three sources and are distributed throughout the body by circulation. From the digestive system the end products of digestion are absorbed in the blood. The respiratory system supplies oxygen. The hormones produced in the endocrine glands are thrown directly into the blood stream. The heart is the chief organ of the circulatory system which pumps the blood through the arteries and their branches, called arterioles. Where the arterioles end the capillaries begin, and they lead next to the veins which return the blood to the heart. In addition to supplying nutrients the blood carries on another important function, that of removal of waste materials from the tissues which are ultimately eliminated through the skin, kidneys, lungs, and the anus.

If a body part is inactive, its blood supply is reduced because the capillaries remain closed and there may be congestion of blood. This means loss of nutrient supply and slow removal of waste materials. Both these conditions lead to a progressive lowering of the efficient working of the part concerned, which may give rise to disorders interfering with the function of that part.

We have already seen how pranayama promotes circulation of blood in the thoracic and abdominal cavities, due to the pressure changes during the different stages of pranayama. This has an influence on the circulation throughout the body. The pressure changes on the heart constitute good exercise to its tissue without putting a load on it. This is one of the most important benefits of pranayama. The state of relaxation characteristic of pranayama is extremely beneficial to heart patients and also to persons of normal health.

In the postures for pranayama the legs are pressed and so less blood flows through them. More blood is therefore available to other parts of the body. This is expected to be helpful in the arousal of the kundalini.

RESPIRATION

The respiratory system is directly influenced by pranayama due to every part of the lungs being filled completely, the walls of the alveoli being stretched and relaxed alternately, due to changes in the ventilatory rate and pressure in the two cavities, and due to the training of the respiratory centre. Pranayama helps to increase the vital capacity and strength of the respiratory muscles. An obvious result of this is more efficient breathing. Cleaning of the respiratory passage is one of the important benefits of pranayama. Due to all these effects pranayama has a great therapeutical value for the treatment of disorders of the respiratory tract. It is one of the best preventive measures in case of these and other disorders.

SECRETION

In our body there are many glands situated at different places which secrete fluids having specific functions. The secretion of a gland is not used in the gland itself. Its function takes place usually at some other place. So the secretion is required to be carried elsewhere. This is done in two ways. Some glands have special passages or ducts to carry the secretion away, e.g., the salivary glands, liver, pancreas, and the gonads. Some glands do dot have any such passages or ducts, and their secretions are thrown directly in the blood stream. They are called endocrine glands. Their secretions, called hormones, govern many vital functions in the body, such as metabolism, growth, action of the heart, blood pressure, sex behaviour, and so on. Excess as well as shortage of the hormones are both detrimental to health. The main endocrine glands are: the pineal and pituitary (in the brain), thyroid and parathyroid (in the neck), thymus (near the heart), adrenals (above the kidneys), and the gonads.

How does pranayama help to keep these glands healthy? The thyroid and parathyroids are pressed in Jalandhara bandha.

The thymus and adrenals are influenced by the pressure changes in the thoracic and abdominal cavities, while the gonads are influenced by Uddiyana bandha and Mula bandha. All these glands are kept healthy by pranayama by exercising their tissue and improving their blood supply.

Influence of pranayama on the pancreas should be specially mentioned here. This gland produces two kinds of fluids. The pancreatic juice which is carried to the duodenum through the pancreatic duct plays an important role in the digestion of food. The other one is a hormone called insulin which is essential for converting glucose into glycogen. Deficiency of this hormone causes diabetes. Pranayama acts as a caretaker of the pancreas, and is therefore very useful in the treatment of diabetes.

EXCRETION

Production of waste materials in the body is a process going on side by side with the process of living. If these waste materials are not removed quickly then they give rise to toxins. Carbon dioxide is one of the most toxic substances which can kill a cell or tissue very quickly. Elimination of waste materials from the body is carried on through the digestive, respiratory, and urinary systems, and also through the skin. All these agencies function well by doing pranayama regularly. The intestines and kidneys benefit in the same way as do the other abdominal viscera, by pressure changes in pranayama and by improvement of circulation. Elimination of carbon dioxide and water vapour has already been discussed at length. Elimination of excess salts in the form of sweat is promoted by pranayama. This is because pranayama stimulates the sweat glands through its influence on the hypothalamus. Any one can experience sweating after a few rounds of pranayama.

Pranayama may thus be called a blood purifier. In traditional texts it is described as the best cleansing procedure for the body and mind, so much so, that for a person practising pranayama regularly it is not necessary to practise any other cleansing technique such as dhauti, basti, and so on.

REPRODUCTION

It is a remarkable characteristic of each species that although each individual belonging to it has a limited span of life, the species itself survives almost indefinitely. This is because each individual is capable of reproducing, and the progeny lives after the individual's life comes to an end. In man the male reproductive system consists of the testes where the sperm is produced, the vas deferens which carries the sperm, the seminal vesicles where the sperm is stored, and the urethra through which it is deposited in the body of the female. The female reproductive system is formed by the ovaries which produce the ova, the oviducts which lead to the uterus, and the uterus where the embryo grows.

Pranayama has a beneficial influence on the organs of reproduction due to pressure changes in the abdominal cavity. Uddiyana bandha and Mula bandha greatly increase this beneficial influence.

CO-ORDINATION OF VARIOUS FUNCTIONS

The human body is an organic whole. No function in it can go on in isolation. Every function is connected with and dependent on many other functions. Co-ordination among the various functions is brought about by the nervous system. It has two parts; (i) the central nervous system, consisting of the brain, the spinal cord, and the spinal nerves, and (ii) the autonomic nervous system. The former governs all the voluntary functions and the latter the involuntary functions. The nervous tissue is highly sensitive to lack of oxygen and excess of carbon dioxide. We have already noted earlier how pranayama, even in a moderate practice, can help to supply enough oxygen and remove carbon dioxide quickly. Kapalabhati is the best exercise for this purpose.

Traditional texts abound in references to the importance of pranayama as a nerve purifier. They have used the term nadi for the nerves, and have spoken of nadishuddhi, i.e., purification of nerves through pranayama and the effects produced by it. The basic idea is that pranayama, by purifying the whole of the nervous system including the brain, ultimately leads to the removal of ignorance and to stability and peace of mind. These are the qualities which everyone of us desires to have but very few do actually possess.

Pranayama may be said to help the coordination of various functions by improving every function and by influencing the nervous system itself. It may thus be called a good body servicing programme which looks after the health of each part and system of the body. It is therefore that pranayama is a key to good health. It improves vitality and flexibility of each organ, especially the vital organs, and thus helps a great deal to increase the power of endurance, both physical and mental.

It may be said in conclusion of this discussion that if one uses this key to good health in time then one can surely enjoy good health and peace of mind throughout the rest of one's life. The earlier one starts using it, the better.

But most of us are apt to forget this fact, and we usually come to do pranayama only when we are compelled by some disorder. What can pranayama do in such cases? We shall discuss this improtant problem in the next chapter.

7

Pranayama
for the Cure of Disorders

The cure of disorders falls actually to the domain of the science of medicine. There has been an awe-inspiring progress in this science over the past quarter century, and due to it man has completely overcome some of the most dreaded diseases of the past such as small pox, cholera, and plague. Half a century ago these diseases and the others such as malaria, influenza, typhoid and tuberculosis used to take a heavy toll of human life. But today not many people die of these diseases. That is certainly due to an increased knowledge of the causes of them and discoveries of powerful means to combat them. But all the progress of medicine has so far unfortunately not led to a healthier human race. Although some diseases are checked, there are others which used to be less common in the days of our ancestors, which are on the increase in our times. For instance, the stress disorders and psychosomatic disorders which were not much heard of one generation before, are now posing a great health hazard. Similarly, disorders due to pollution, crowding, lack of exercise and faulty food habits are much more common now as compared to the past.

It is not that medicine is totally helpless or ineffective against these disorders. But the trouble is that the cure which the science of medicine offers is in many cases temporary. So the disorder continues in spite of medication. This has led people to think of other means of cure, such as Ayurvedic medicine, Nature Cure, and Homoeopathy. The most recent addition to the list of these other means is Yoga. Its techniques have become popular recently mainly because they seem to offer lasting relief in case of some disorders where medicines fail. Another strong point about the yoga techniques is that they are not expensive. Moreover, they are useful for the maintenance of general or overall health apart from removing particular disorders. It is in this context that we shall discuss in this chapter how pranayama can be applied for the cure of some common and chronic disorders.

The first point to be noted about the therapeutic application of pranayama is the well known saying "prevention is better than cure". The preventive value of pranayama is much more important than its curative value. We have already mentioned the fact earlier that one should learn the techniques of pranayama much before one is overtaken by a disorder so that the disorder does not develop at all, or if it does, then its severity is reduced because the general strength and vitality of the system concerned is increased by practising pranayama. Of course, it is not the case that every disorder can be prevented or checked by pranayama. In fact there is no such panacea in existence. Even modern medicine with all its life saving drugs and powerful techniques cannot hold such a claim. But it is found by many a consulting physician that pranayama does a marvellous job in our fight against some of the diseases. If more and more people become aware of this fact and take to the practice of pranayama at the earliest opportunity then we shall all be living in a much healthier and thus happier world.

But howsoever this may be true, it is a fact that most of us turn to pranayama only as a last resort, when medicine fails to give enough relief. One advantage peculiar to medicines is that if a medicine works then one does not have to do anything further by oneself, i.e., one does not have to exert, because the job of curing the disorder is done solely by the drug. That is not the case with nature cure or yoga or pranayama, where one has to go through some tedious procedures. So it is natural for every one to try the drugs first and it is only if they fail that one remembers other methods. Due to this tendency of people to begin learning pranayama when a disease threatens to go out of hand in spite of taking drugs, it becomes difficult to draw the fullest benefit from pranayama.

Cause of ill health

Before we consider how pranayama can be applied as a curative measure in the case of particular disorders it would be better to consider various conditions which lead to ill health, because unless those conditions are removed any curative technique will not work effectively. Among such causes we may list environmental conditions, heredity, lack of moderation of behaviour, faulty diet, imbalance between work and rest, pollution, cleanliness and hygiene, lack of exercise, and stress and strain. Let us see how each one of these factors contributes to ill heath so that before practising pranayama for the cure of illness one may also try to remove the factors causing it.

Environmental conditions

We are hardly ever aware of the role the environment plays in health and illness because we usually live in more or less congenial environmental conditions. For a healthy living it is necessary that there should not be too wide variations in heat and cold, humidity and dryness, atmospheric pressure and presence of oxygen. There should be no lethal gases in the atmosphere. Non-availability of clean drinking water becomes a limiting factor for health. Enough open air is an important factor for health. In some disorders such as allergy, asthma, dysentery, dyspepsia and headache, a change of weather helps a great deal. People suffering from constipation and gastric troubles often find that variations in drinking water have considerable effect on their ailments. Soft water helps to reduce these troubles, while hard water which contains inorganic salts is bad for digestion.

Heredity

Out of the characteristics one possesses some are acquired in response to the environment, while some are inherited. For instance, sustained use of the muscles builds them up, while the muscles which are not used atrophy. The acquired characteristics are not transmitted from one generation to another. A child of blind parents need not be blind. Qualities like eye colour, skin colour, colour blindness, baldness, and diseases like asthma, diabetes, and obesity show influence of hereditary factors. Individuals whose parents have these disorders are therefore well advised to start doing pranayama at an early age so as to overcome the proneness to these disorders.

There is a good deal of interaction between heredity and environment giving rise to individual variations. Thus it is often found that out of the children of asthmatic or diabetic parents some may suffer and others may not. Thus although one may be born with a kind of proneness to a certain disease one can improve the resistance to it by doing pranayama and thus escape an onset of the disease. Of course, this has its limitations, but every one can expect to get some relief if the practice of pranayama is started well in time.

Moderation of behaviour

In daily life every one of us has to do various activities such as work and rest, eating food, meeting people, and so on. A moderation of these various activities is essential for good health. Taking exercise, eating food, sleeping, working, and meeting people are all good and desirable things. Similarly, entertainment and enjoyment is also necessary for every one of us. But if any of these activities is carried to its extreme, for instance, if we eat too much, or work or sleep or talk too much then it will certainly have a bad effect on health. On the other hand, having too little of rest or food or enjoyment would also influence health adversely. This is true of the habits of drinking, smoking and enjoying sex also. One should learn to adjust one's behaviour at an equal distance from 'too much' and 'too little'. This is perhaps a golden rule to be followed for enjoying good health.

This is, indeed, quite easy to understand, but rather difficult to follow. There are many people who suffer from ill health not due to hereditary factors or infection or a chronic disease, but mainly due to carelessness and ignorance of the importance of moderation of behaviour. Such persons can get sufficient relief simply by changing their pattern of behaviour in daily life. In addition to this, if they do pranayama they may certainly enjoy good health. Lack of moderation of behaviour is an enemy of good health.

Faulty diet

We have already discussed the yoga view of balanced diet, according to which what we eat should satisfy the needs of the body. Many of us suffer either from malnutrition or from excess of nutrition. What we digest and assimilate is more important than what we eat. It is of little use if one takes a rich and nutritious diet while one has no power of digesting it properly. Eating energy-rich substances without doing much work results into accumulation of fat in the body. Eating too many times, too much at one time, too much of spices and fats, or taking too much of fried food, eating in a hurry, are some of the common mistakes which make the diet faulty. Faulty diet aggravates disorders, and may itself be the cause of some disorders.

Imbalance between work and rest

Both work and rest are necessary for human life. More work and no rest is bad for health. Similarly, more rest and no work is also not congenial to good health. Both should be properly balanced. Without proper rest the muscles and nerves may wear out. But without proper work they become dull and lose their efficiency. There should also be a balance between mental and physical work.

Cleanliness and hygiene

Bodily hygiene and cleanliness is essential for good health. Social hygiene is also equally important. Mental hygiene is perhaps even more important than these two. The idea of cleanliness in most of us is limited to the body and the clothes. Cleanliness of the surroundings and that of the mind are also important constituents of individual and social health. Neglect of these often leads to ill health. Lack of cleanliness in kitchens and utensils, especially where many people eat together, is a potent source of spread of diseases of the gastro-intestinal tract.

Pollution

This has developed into an acute problem everywhere in cities and industrial towns. Presence of smoke and gaseous bye-products of industries in the atmosphere of towns is detrimental to health. There is pollution due to improper disposal of sewage water. Pollution of drinking water causes water borne diseases on a large scale. Pollution due to crowding is also a difficult problem faced by growing cities. Adulteration of food, milk, medicines, and drugs must also be considered as bad as pollution of the atmosphere or even sometimes more dangerous so far as the health of the individual and society is concerned. Pollution due to nuclear explosions can prove to be the deadliest among the sources of pollution in the future. All these forms of pollution are ravaging the human society in the present age of scientific progress and industrial and technological growth.

Lack of exercise

Among all the causes of common disorders the one single cause which contributes to them much than others is perhaps lack of exercise. Inertia or inaction seems to be a universal characteristic of matter. This characteristic expresses itself in the world of living beings in the form "not to move unless compelled to move" This is true even of activities such as thinking. Just as economy of expenditure is a natural tendency, so is the tendency of economy of movement or economy of exertion. Thus taking regular exercise is somewhat against man's nature. It is only those who become aware of the possible loss of health if exercise is not taken, that exert themselves physically by doing exercise.

In the absence of exercise the muscles and joints slowly lose their strength and efficiency. Fat may start accumulating if the intake of calories is more than their expenditure. Efficiency of various functions is also reduced slowly. Blood circulation is not promoted. Vitality, endurance and resistance to diseases may be lowered in the long run, and so disorders due to sluggishness of vital organs start making their appearance. Of course it is not the case that those who take regular exercise

Asanas for Healing

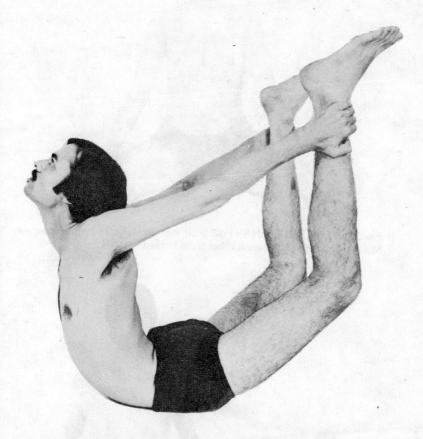

Fig. 30 : DHANURASANA : The body is turned like a bow. It stretches the abdominal muscles and the back.

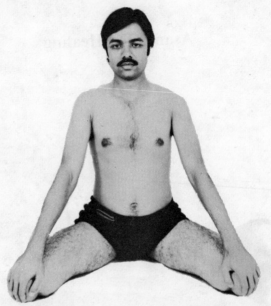

Fig. 31 : MANDUKASANA : Fold your legs and take an angular posture. Make your heels touch each other from behind.

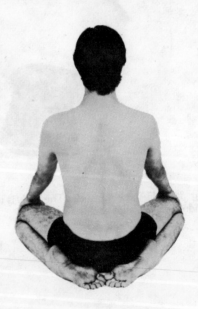

Fig. 32 : Back View

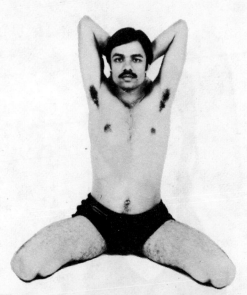

Fig. 33 : UTTANA MANDUKASANA : Take the posture of mandukasana. Fold your hands and hold them crossed touching your elbows by the palms.

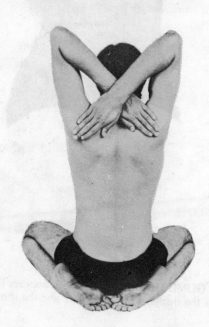

Fig. 34 : Back View

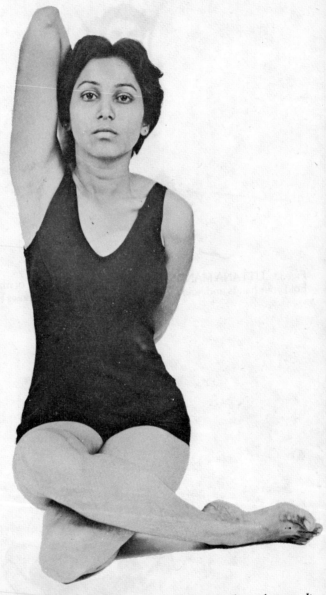

Fig. 35 : GOMUKHASANA : The body appears like the face of a cow. It exercises the thighs, lower abdomen, and the shoulders.

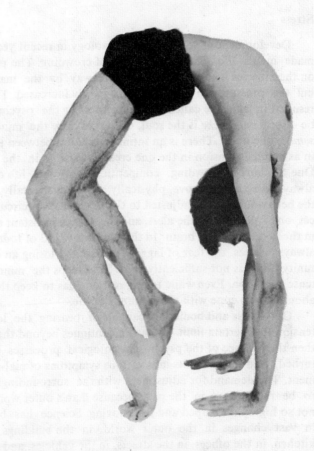

Fig. 36 : CHAKRASANA : The body is made to appear like a wheel. Provides good stretching exercise to almost all the skeletal muscles.

are completely free of disorders only because they exercise their bodies. But it is true also that by taking regular exercise one can eliminate a very formidable cause of disorders. One who takes exercise regularly is definitely better placed in fighting the other causes also, such as environmental conditions, pollution, etc.

Stress

Development of science and technology in recent years has made man's life fast, busy and full of crowding. The pressure on the muscles has been largely taken away by the machines, but the pressure on the nerves has greatly increased. This has resulted in what are called stress disorders or the psychosomatic disorders. *Psyche* is the soul, or let us say the mind, and *soma* is the body. There is an intimate relation between the two in as much as tension in the one creates tension in the other. Due to hurry, crowding, competition, and fast life one has always to be on the move, physically as well as mentally. When the behaviour is to be adjusted to the demands of circumstances one has to be on the alert, and this creates constant tension in the nerves and the brain. In the complex world of today, one always carries the fear of lagging behind and losing an opportunity if one is not sufficiently alert. This keeps the mind in a tense condition. Even while taking rest one has to keep thinking about how to cope with the demands of life.

Our minds and bodies are capable of bearing the load of tension to a certain limit. If tension continues beyond that limit then the balance of the psycho-physiological processes is disturbed, and that results into various symptoms of mal-adjustment. The demand for adjustment with the surroundings used to be rather low in the past, because man's outer world was not so highly developed and fast moving. Science has brought in vast changes in the outer world, in the buildings, in the kitchen, in the offices, in the streets, in the vehicles, and in the various gadgets and instruments of daily use. Adjustment of behaviour with this complex and demanding outer world is far more difficult than what it used to be half a century ago. Need to adjust inevitably gives rise to tension.

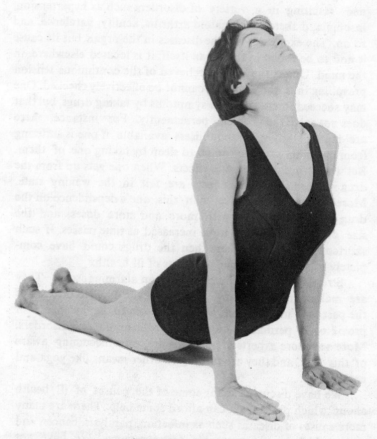

Fig. 37 : BHUJANGASANA : Bend backward the neck and the back causing
extension of the spine. The navel is not to be raised. Good for a healthy
spine.

Tension in the mind expresses itself in the form of impulses that flow from the brain to various muscles of the body, such as the facial muscles, muscles of the forehead and neck, those of the abdominal wall and the smooth muscles of the internal organs. If these impulses continue to make an impact on the glands and organs, they interfere with their normal functioning. This gives rise to malfunctioning of the organ or gland concerned, resulting in a variety of disorders such as hypertension, insomnia, diabetes, rheumatoid arthritis, acidity, flatulence, and so on. The expression of the diseases in the organ, but its cause is not to be found in the organ itself; it is located elsewhere, in the mind. Unless the mind is relieved of the continuous tension prevailing in it, the disorder cannot be effectively checked. One may succeed in checking the symptoms by taking drugs, but that does not solve the problem permanently. For instance, there are many kinds of tranquillisers available if one is suffering from insomnia and one can go to sleep by taking one of them. But the drugs do have side effects. When one gets up from the drug induced sleep these effects are felt in the waking state. Moreover, what is worse than this, one's dependence on the drug goes on increasing with more and more doses, and the size of the dose is also to be increased as time passes. If such shortcomings were not there then the drugs could have completely solved many of our problems of ill health.

Stress disorders are increasing on an alarming scale. They are making man's victory on some of the dreaded diseases of the past look insignificant. Medicines seem to be incapable of providing a permanent cure of the problem of stress disorders. More and more experts of medicine are now becoming aware of this fact, and they are turning to other means like yoga and nature cure.

We have discussed so far some of the causes of ill health about which pranayama can afford some help. There are many more causes of diseases such as infection, paralysis, cancer, and so on, which are not amenable to pranayama. We have not considered these causes here. It is not our contention that pranayama can cure all the diseases. Indeed, pranayama is not a substitute to medicine. It has only a small jurisdiction in therapy. It does not and cannot cover the whole field of therapy. This is an important fact which every student and

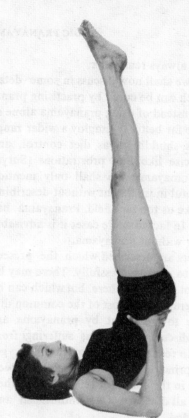

Fig. 38 : VIPARITA-KARANI : The legs are held together in an inverted position. The back makes an angle of 45 degrees with the ground. Promotes venous blood circulation.

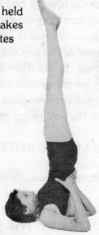

Fig. 39 : SARVANGASANA : The back is held straight, up-side down. The chin touches the chest below the throat. Improves the function of the thyroid.

teacher of pranayama must always remember.

Remembering this fact we shall now discuss in some detail the various disorders which can be cured by practising pranayama. In most of the cases instead of using pranayama alone as a relief measure it would be far better to employ a wider range of techniques such as asanas, shuddhi kriyas, diet control, and more active form of exercise like Sun prostrations (Suryanamaskara) in addition to pranayama. We shall only mention these other techniques useful in treatment without describing them because that would take us too far afield. Pranayama has no antagonism to medicine. In fact in acute cases it is advisable to take medical help with or without pranayama.

Here only those disorders are described which the present writer has had a chance to treat successfully. There may be other disorders which are not mentioned here, but which can be treated with pranayama therapy. But most of the common disorders which are amenable to treatment by pranayama are covered in the following discussion. Persons suffering from these disorders are advised to read the discussion carefully, get acquainted with the basic principles involved which have been described at different places in the course of this book, and then start doing pranayama with all due care. Over-enthusiasm and haste should always be avoided.

Disorders may be classified according to the system involved, such as disorders of the gastro-intestinal tract, respiratory tract, those of the circulatory, nervous or urino-genital system, and so on. Some disorders do not affect any particular system and may be connected with more than one systems. They may be grouped under general disorders. We shall discuss the disorders in the following order:

GENERAL DISORDERS

Postural defects, headache, migraine, backache, diabetes, obesity.

DISORDERS OF THE GASTRO-INTESTINAL TRACT

Constipation, flatulence, dyspepsia, acidity, ulcers, chronic dysentery, piles.

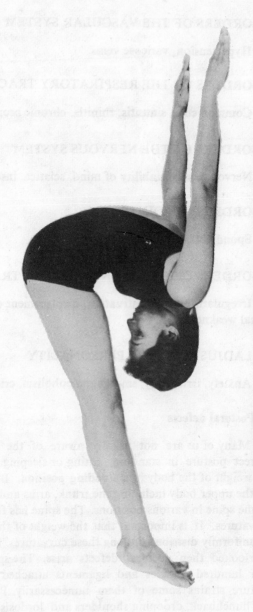

Fig. 40 : HALASANA : The feet are kept behind the head, without bending the legs at the knees. It gives good exercise to the back.

DISORDERS OF THE VASCULAR SYSTEM

Hypertension, varicose veins.

DISORDERS OF THE RESPIRATORY TRACT

Common cold, sinusitis, rhinitis, chronic bronchitis, asthma.

DISORDERS OF THE NERVOUS SYSTEM

Nervousness, instability of mind, sciatica, insomnia.

DISORDERS OF JOINTS

Spondylitis, arthritis, gout.

DISORDERS OF THE URINO-GENITAL TRACT

Irregularities of menstruation, displacement of the uterus, sexual weakness.

MALADJUSTMENT OF PERSONALITY

Anxiety, irritability, smoking, alcoholism, criminality.

1. Postural defects

Many of us are not usually aware of the importance of correct posture in standing, sitting or sleeping. The legs bear the weight of the body in a standing position. But the weight of the upper body including the trunk, arms and head is borne by the spine in various positions. The spine has four arches or curvatures. It is important that the weight of the body should be uniformly distributed along these curvatures. If this fact is overlooked then postural defects arise. The spine has nearly four hundred muscles and ligaments attached to it. Faulty posture strains some of them unnecessarily. Postural defects like hunchback, drooping shoulders and lordosis are common among more than half of the population. These defects in the long run give rise to pain in the back, shoulders and neck,

SHIRSHASANA

FIRST STAGE

SECOND STAGE

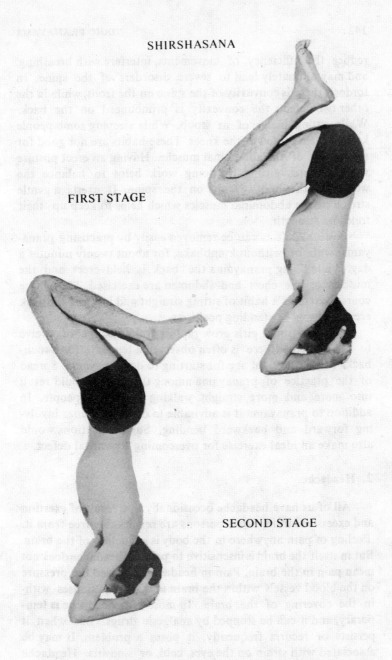

Fig. 41, 42 & 43 : SHIRSHASANA : The body is held straight, up-side down, on the head. It promotes circulation and removes congestion of blood.

reduce the efficiency of movements, interfere with breathing, and may ultimately lead to severe disorders of the spine. In lordosis there is convexity of the spine on the front, while in the other two defects the convexity is pronounced on the back. While sitting many of us stoop. While sleeping some people keep the legs folded at the knees. These habits are not good for the health of the abdominal muscles. Having an erect posture while standing, sitting or doing work helps to balance the weight of the body evenly on the spine. It exerts a gentle stretch on the abdominal muscles which helps to keep up their tone and strength.

Postural defects can be removed easily by practising prana-yama with or without kumbhaka, for about twenty minutes a day. While doing pranayama the back is held erect and the muscles of the chest and abdomen are exercised. This in due course generates a habit of sitting straight and keeping the back erect in sitting or standing positions.

When boys and girls grow rapidly from the age of twelve to fifteen years there is often observed a tendency for hunch-back. This is the right age for starting to do pranayama. Spread of the practice of pranayama among the masses would result into more and more straight walking and erect people. In addition to pranayama it is advisable to do some asanas involv-ing forward and backward bending. Sun prostrations would also make an ideal exercise for overcoming a postural defect.

2. Headache

All of us have headache occasionally as a result of exertion and excessive strain. Some persons are remarkably free from it. Feeling of pain anywhere in the body is a function of the brain. But in itself the brain is insensitive to pain. So headache does not mean pain in the brain. Pain in headache is caused by pressure on the blood vessels within the brain and venous sinuses with-in the covering of the brain. In most cases headache is tem-porary, and it can be stopped by analgesic drugs. But when it persists or recurrs frequently, it poses a problem. It may be associated with strain on the eyes, cold, or sinusitis. Headache due to meningeal involvement is very severe.

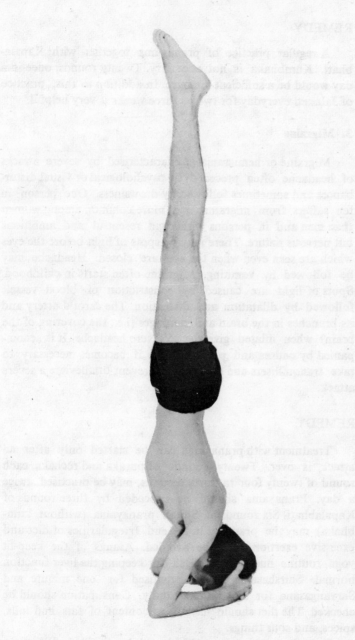

FINAL STAGE

REMEDY

A regular practice of pranayama together with Kapalabhati. Kumbhaka is not necessary. Twenty rounds, once in a
day would be a sufficient measure. In addition to this, practice
of Jalaneti everyday for two to three weeks is very helpful.

3. Migraine

Migraine or hemicrania is characterised by severe attacks
of headache often preceded by psychological or visual disturbances and sometimes followed by drowsiness. One person in
ten suffers from migraine. It is more common among women
than men and in persons with rigid resentful and ambitious
but nervous nature. There may be spots of light before the eyes
which are seen even when the eyes are closed. Headache may
be followed by vomiting. Migraine often starts in childhood.
Spots of light are caused by constriction of blood vessels
followed by dilatation and distention. The carotid artery and
its branches in the brain and meninges (i.e., the covering of the
brain) when dilated give rise to severe headache. It is accompanied by nausea and photophobia. It becomes necessary to
take tranquillisers and sedatives to prevent or alleviate a severe
attack.

REMEDY

Treatment with pranayama can be started only after an
attack is over. Twenty rounds of puraka and rechaka, each
round of twenty four to thirty seconds, may be practised twice
a day. Pranayama should be preceded by three rounds of
Kapalabhati. Six rounds of Shitali pranayama (without kumbhaka) may be practised in the end. Irregularities of diet and
excessive exertion must be avoided. Asanas of the keep-fit
yoga routine may be practised for keeping the liver function
normal. Shirshasana may be practised for one minute and
Sarvangasana for five minutes daily. Constipation should be
checked. The diet should have low content of fats and oils,
spices, and sour things.

Exposure to heat or cold should be avoided. When an

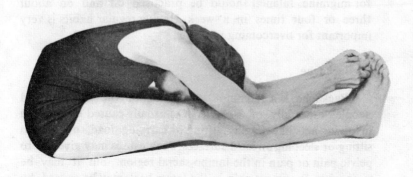

Fig. 44 : PASCHIMOTTANASANA : The fore-head is placed on the knees without raising the latter. Exerts a pull on the spine, and pressure on the abdominal viscera.

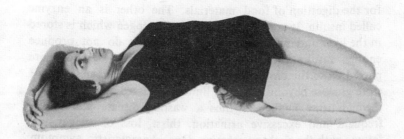

Fig. 45 : SUPTA VAJRASANA : After doing Vajrasana (see p. 51), one lies down on the back. It is very useful in removing constipation

attack of migraine is expected one should relax after a warm bath in a darkened room. Practice of neti is a very good remedy for migraine. Jalaneti should be practised off and on about three or four times in a week. Having regular habits is very important for overcoming migraine.

4. Backache

Backache is a common complaint of the middle aged people, especially of women. It is usually caused by exertion involving acts like digging, lifting or carrying load, or due to sitting or sleeping on hard surfaces. Such causes may give rise to pelvic pain or pain in the lumbo-sacral region. But it may be temporary. Persistent pain in the lower back may be caused by lack of exercise, congestion of blood, or infection of the kidneys or uterus. The cause should be diagnosed by medical investigation, and if there is no infection then pranayama can provide the best remedial measure.

5. Diabetes

Diabetes is a disorder which may be inherited. All the children of parents (either or both) having diabetes may not show it, but it can appear after a gap of a generation. Diabetes is caused by a deficiency of function of the pancreas which is a tongue-shaped organ placed in the abdominal cavity, behind the stomach. It produces two secretions. One is the pancreatic juice which is carried to the duodenum by the pancreatic duct for the digestion of food materials. The other is an enzyme called insulin. It converts glucose into glycogen which is stored in the liver and in the tissues. If the pancreas do not produce enough insulin then abnormally large quantities of glucose are passed on to the blood. Since the blood and the tissues cannot store glucose beyond a certain limit it is passed out of the body through urine. Diabetes is thus a wasting disease marked by frequent and excessive urination, thirst, loss of weight, and fatigue with the slightest exertion. One characteristic symptom is slow healing of wounds. One feels hungry most of the time and the weight goes on reducing in spite of eating much food, because of elimination of glucose from the kidneys which in

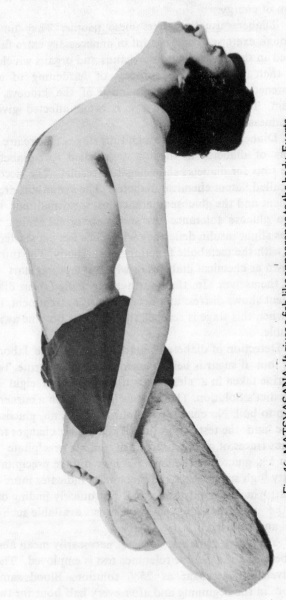

Fig. 46: MATSYASANA : It gives a fish-like appearance to the body. Exerts a stretch on the abdominal wall, throat and the back muscles.

normal people is used for oxidation in the tissues for production of energy.

Diabetes usually prefers obese people. They do not take enough exercise. There is a lot of unnecessary extra fat accumulated in the body around the glands and organs which decreases their efficiency. The process of hardening of arteries is hastened. This may result in damage of the kidneys, heart or brain. The retina of the eye is often affected giving rise to blindness in severe cases.

Diabetes proceeds through four stages. There are no symptoms of diabetes in the first stage called 'pre-diabetic phase.' The tests for diabetes show negative results. The second stage is called 'latent chemical diabetes.' The symptoms are not very evident and the glucose tolerance test is normal, but the cortisone glucose tolerance test shows abnormal results. This indicates slight insulin deficiency which has not yet started interfering with the metabolic functions of the body. The third stage is known as chemical diabetes in which symptoms start manifesting themselves. In the fourth stage called overt diabetes the patient shows distress and need for insulin treatment. It is usually when this stage is reached that patients become aware of the trouble.

Detection of diabetes is made by tests in the laboratory to find out if sugar is being passed through the urine. To five ml. of urine taken in a clean test-tube are added eight drops of Benedict's Solution. This mixture is heated on a burner or spirit lamp to boil, No change of colour indicates no glucose in the urine and the test is negative. If the colour changes to green it means traces of glucose. Greenish yellow precipitate indicates upto 1% glucose in the urine. Yellow orange precipitate means pretty high sugar. Brick red precipitate indicates more than 2% sugar, which is highly abnormal. For quickly finding out sugar in the urine there are some quick tests available such as 'clinitest' and 'clinistix'.

A negative urine test does not necessarily mean absence of diabetes. So the glucose tolerance test is employed. The patient is given 100 gm. sugar as 25% solution. Blood samples are taken in the beginning and after every half hour for two hours. The glucose content of the blood is estimated. Normally the blood contains 60 to 100 mg. of glucose per 100 ml. of blood.

Fig. 47 : SHALABHASANA : Lying down on the chest both the legs are raised together. It exercises the lower back and the abdominal muscles.

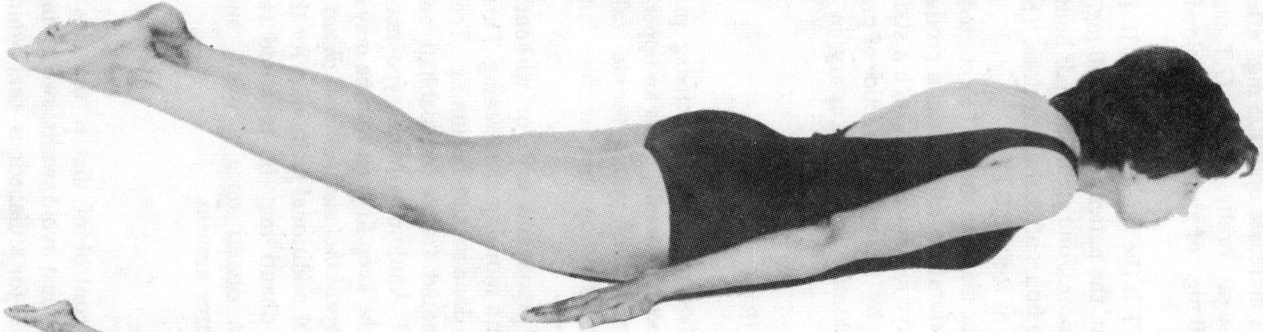

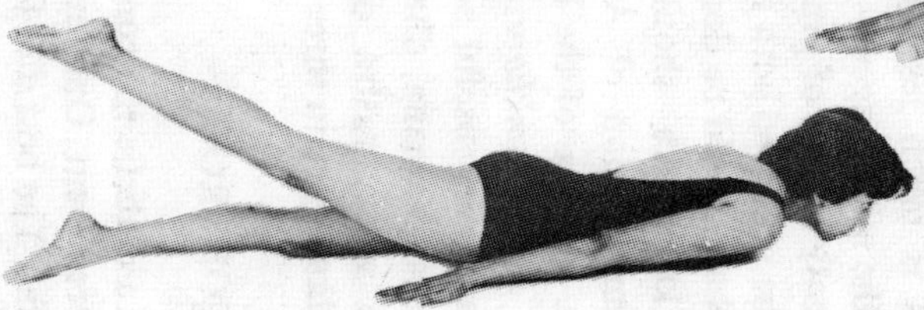

Fig. 48 : ARDHA SHALABHASANA : Only one leg is raised at a time, stretching it backward.

In normal persons this increases upto 125 mg. after two hours of taking 100 gm. sugar orally. In the G.T. test if a patient shows higher than 140 mg. of glucose in the blood that is an indication of diabetes.

The cortisone GTT is the surest test of all. It is similar to the GTT except that the patient is given 50 mg. of cortisone acetate orally in two doses, one eight and half hours before the test and the other two hours after the first dose. The rest of the procedure is the same as for the GTT.

It is important that diabetes should be detected at an early stage when the deterioration of the insulin producing cells of the pancreas might have just started. At such a state it can be very well controlled by a regular practice of pranayama. In later stages insulin treatment may be necessary in addition to pranayama.

REMEDIAL MEASURES

Would be diabetics must start practising pranayama as early as possible. Diabetes generally gains an upper hand in the latter half of life. Diabetes of young people, called juvenile diabetes is much less common, but far more dangerous than that of the middle aged.

Twenty rounds of pranayama with or without kumbhaka should be practised both morning and evening. Three rounds of kapalabhati should be done in the beginning. Ten rounds of bahya kumbhaka should follow kapalabhati and then the pranayama session of Anuloma-viloma type may be gone through. Asanas of the keep fit yoga routine may be practised once a day. *Shankhaprakshalana, vamana dhauti* and *vastra dhauti* are very useful additional techniques for the treatment of diabetes. Vamana dhauti may be practised two or three times a week, vastra dhauti once a week, and shankha prakshalana once in three months.

DIET CONTROL

For a diabetic the control of diet is the most important part of treatment. One must avoid sweets, sweet fruits, eggs and animal fat. The best diet for a diabetic is that which contains

Surya Namaskara

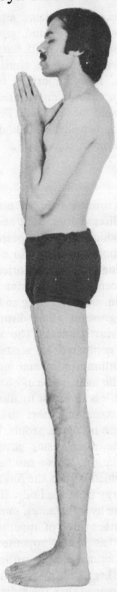

Position 1 : Stand erect and fold your hands.

Fig. 49 to 58 : SURYA NAMASKARA : Though not included in Hatha Yoga techniques, it is very good for health and very popular all over India. It involves various postures, bending forward and backward. If practised regularly before doing yogic postures and pranayama, it can prove to be an excellent caretaker of health.

152

YOGIC PRANAYAMAYOGIC PRANAYAMA

40% carbohydrates, 15% proteins and 45% fats. One should include enough raw vegetables and green leafy vegetables in the daily diet. One may take milk but not potatoes, sugar and starchy foods. Obesity must be considered an equally bad enemy as diabetes. It is important to take enough fluids for keeping the function of the kidneys normal. Constipation and mental tension should be avoided. Practice of meditation to keep tensions away is beneficial. Meditation may be practised while doing pranayama or separately.

6. Obesity

In itself obesity is not a disorder. But it often incapacitates a person just as a disease does. So it needs correction. Because there are no drugs which can help a person to lose extra fat and one has to exert both mentally for not eating too much and physically for burning the excess calories, the obese people find it very difficult to keep the body trim. We often hear them complaining that in spite of eating so little their weight is not reduced. Obesity aggravates other disorders such as diabetes mellitus, gout, and heart ailments. The obese are more prone to catch infection as compared to persons of normal weight. Obesity increases both morbidity and mortality.

Over-eating is the main cause of obesity. This we all know very well. But to eat less so as not to allow extra fat to accumulate in the body is something next to impossible. Otherwise there would have been no obese people. Usually in us there is a balance between the mechanisms governing the feelings of hunger and its satiation. These mechanisms are governed by the hypothalamus which adjusts the food intake to the level of expenditure of energy from the body. It is supposed that there are two centres in the hypothalamus, one controlling reactions of satiety and the other those of appetite. It has been observed in case of animals that if the appetite controlling centre is damaged then the animal stops eating and may even die of starvation. On the other hand, if the centre controlling satiety becomes weak or damaged then the animal goes on eating.

In some cases over-eating may be caused by unconscious emotional disturbances. Substitute for gratification is supplied by over-eating when one has despair, anguish, and repression of

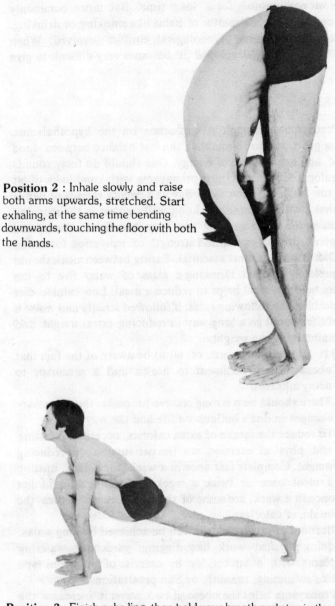

Position 2 : Inhale slowly and raise both arms upwards, stretched. Start exhaling, at the same time bending downwards, touching the floor with both the hands.

Position 3 : Finish exhaling, then hold your breath and stay in the position for a few seconds. Then put both the hands on the floor, raising the head and stretching the left leg backwards.

emotions continuously for a long time. But more commonly over-eating is just a matter of habit like smoking or drinking. There may be no inner psychological conflict involved. When once the habit is developed it becomes very difficult to give it up.

REMEDY

Pranayama, through its influence on the hypothalamus, helps a great deal to re-establish the lost balance between food intake and expenditure of energy. One should do forty rounds of Anuloma-viloma or Ujjayi pranayama with kumbhaka of at least ten seconds once in a day and twenty rounds of bahya kumbhaka with the bandhas. Long walks either in the morning or evening for about an hour are very beneficial. Pranayama also gives the will power and strength of resolution for eating less. Diet control is most essential. Eating between meals should be completely stopped. Drinking a glass of water five to ten minutes before a meal helps to reduce a meal. Low calorie diet is advisable. The following rules, if followed strictly and made a part of life, would go a long way in reducing extra weight and then maintaining the weight.

(i) It is necesssary first of all to be aware of the fact that obesity is an impediment to health and a precursor to many ailments.

(ii) There should be a strong resolve to make the necessary changes in one's outlook on life and the way of life.

(iii) To reduce the intake of extra calories, occasional fasting and physical exertion are the two sure ways of reducing weight. Complete fast once in a week (for a day), missing a meal once or twice a week, and having a liquid diet once in a week, are some of the measures to reduce the intake of calories.

(iv) Burning of excess calories can be achieved by long walks, doing physical work like digging, gardening, watering plants with a bucket, or by exercise of a rigorous type like swimming, running, or Sun prostrations.

(v) Pranayama helps the obese it two ways: it increases the strength of mind and reduces tensions, and it has an

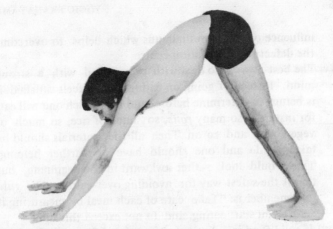

Position 4 : Stretch the right leg too and raise the body.

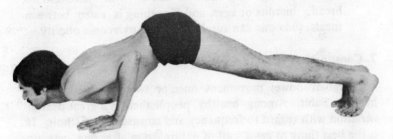

Position 5 : Perform a *danda* by lowering your chest, touching the floor with your chin.

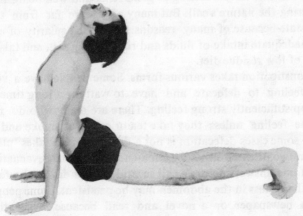

Position 6 : Raise your head, trunk, hips, thighs and knees from the floor.

influence on the hypothalamus which helps to overcome the defect in the satiation centre.

(vi The best way is to deal with every meal with a strong mind. Instead of going on eating till one feels satisfied it is better to determine beforehand how much one will eat, for instance so many *rotis*, so much of rice, so much of vegetables, and so on. Then all the materials should be taken aside, and one should have no further helping. This would look rather awkward in the beginning, but that is the safest way for avoiding over-eating. The rule to remember is: "Take care of each meal by measuring it before you start eating, and do not exceed this limit."

(vi) If solid food is eliminated from breakfast and afternoon snacks, taking only milk or tea or fruit juice and no bread, biscuits or eggs, and if nothing is eaten between meals, then one can surely expect to overcome obesity.

7. Constipation

Regular bowel movement once or twice every day is a healthy habit. Among healthy people there is a great deal of variation with regard to frequency and consistency of stools. It is the best thing to get a 'call of nature' soon after one gets up in the morning, to finish the act of defecation in just a few minutes and to have a feeling of good relief and well being after answering the nature's call. But many of us are far from this ideal state because of many reasons such as irregularity of eating, inadequate intake of fluids and roughage in diet, and taking much of low residue diet.

Constipation takes various forms. Some people have a very mild feeling to defecate and have to wait for a long time to develop sufficiently strong feeling. There are many who do not get the feeling unless they take tea or coffee or smoke and so on. In some cases defecation is not a daily affair; it takes place once in two or three days. There may not be complete evacuation even if one answers nature's call several times a day, and a feeling of heaviness in the abdomen may be persistent. Some people take a newspaper or a novel and read because evacuation takes a very long time. And a few of us have to depend on lax-

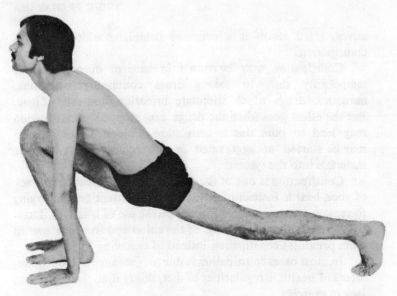

Position 7 : The right foot is brought forward and the left leg is stretched back.

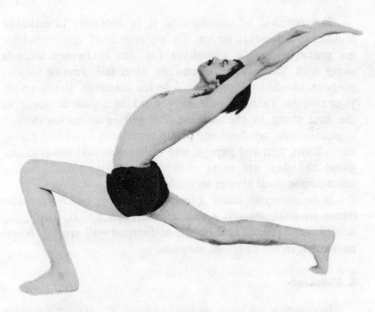

Position 8 : Raise the body with hands in the air.

atives. Hard stools is a common complaint which goes with
constipation.

Constipation may be caused in case of normal persons
temporarily due to taking drugs containing belladona,
narcotics, drugs which stimulate urination, and salts of iron.
But the effect goes when the drugs are stopped. Constipation
may lead to piles due to congestion of blood. Other ailments
may be started or aggravated due to re-absorption of toxic
materials into the system.

Constipation is one of the most common indications of lack
of good health. Instead of giving it serious attention and trying
to remove its cause many of us rely on the use of laxatives. Laxatives irritate the inner lining of the colon and frequent use of
them promotes constipation instead of removing it.

In most cases constipation is due to ignorance of the requirements of health, irregularities of diet, faulty diet, laziness, and
lack of exercise.

REMEDY

For removal of constipation it is necessary to make the
muscles of defecation strong. Twenty rounds of Anuloma-viloma pranayama with kumbhaka for ten to twenty seconds
along with the bandhas forms on ideal daily routine for this
purpose. In addition, one should do the asanas of the keep fit
yoga routine. Taking a walk daily, drinking a glass of water as
the first thing in the morning after getting up, eating enough
vegetables and raw food and pectin containing fruits like guava,
citrus fruits, figs, and papaya, and drinking enough fluids throughout the day, are some of the points which persons having
constipation must always remember.

It is observed many a time that drinking lukewarm water
(three to four glasses) with a little salt added to it, then doing
Suptavajrasana, and rubbing the abdominal wall sets in bowel
movement in ten to fifteen minutes.

8. Flatulence

In common parlance we hear so much about gastric trouble
which is a popular name of flatulence. It is a widespread com-

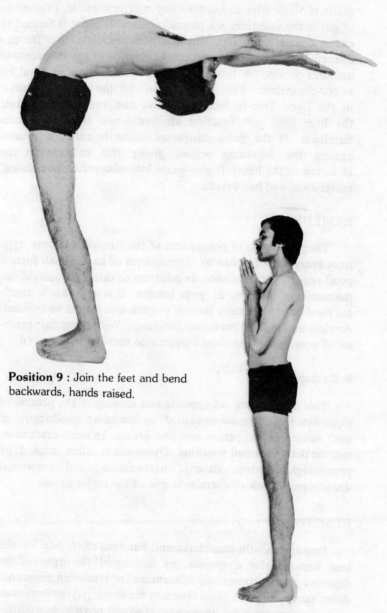

Position 9 : Join the feet and bend
backwards, hands raised.

Position 10 : Return to the original position and stand erect.

plaint of those who do not take any regular exercise. Formation
of gas in the intestines is a natural process. When it is formed in
excess it poses a problem. The intestines absorb some of the gas
formed during digestion of food. Formation of gas in excessive
amounts is due to fermentation or putrifaction of food by
micro-organisms. This is checked by the bile produced
in the liver. Due to lack of exercise and faulty food habits
the liver does not function efficiently, and that results into
flatulence. If the gas is obstructed inside the colon, it presses
against the adjoining organs, giving rise to pain in the
abdomen or the heart. It may cause loss of appetite, uneasiness,
indigestion, and bad breath.

REMEDY

Twenty rounds of pranayama of the Anuloma-viloma type
once every day preceded by three rounds of kapalabhati form a
good remedy for flatulence. In addition to this one should do
the asanas of the keep fit yoga routine. It is imporant to regul-
ate food habits. A heavy fat and protein diet should be avoided.
Anxiety and tension promotes flatulence. With a regular practice of pranayama one should overcome tensions in the mind.

9. Dyspepsia

This means lack of appetite and slowing of the process of
digestion. It is often accompanied by excessive production of
gas, nausea, constipation and foul breath. In some cases there
may be diarrhoea and vomiting. Dyspepsia is often caused by
psychological stress, anxeity, nervousness, and emotional
disturbances. Lack of exercise is one of the major causes.

REMEDY

Pranayama with kumbhaka and bandhas offers one of the
best remedies for dyspepsia, by making all the organs of the
digestive system strong and efficient and by removing emotional
disturbances from the mind. One may practise Ujjayi or Anuloma-
viloma pranayama. Practising asanas would provide an additional advantage. Agnisara is a very helpful technique of yoga for

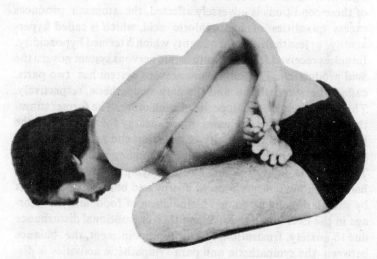

Fig. 59 : YOGA MUDRA : After doing Padmasana (see page 49) one bends forward, keeping the forehead on the ground. It presses the abdominal viscera and stretches the back muscles.

overcoming weakness of digestion. It consists of moving the abdominal wall backward and forward in a standing position, keeping the hands on the knees and bending the body slightly forward. The breath is held out while moving the wall of the abdomen. Taking enough B Complex vitamins is important.

10. Acidity

The inner lining of the stomach secretes hydrochloric acid which plays an important role in digestion. The secretion of this acid by the stomach is influenced by many factors such as presence of food in the stomach, condition of the stomach wall, sight and smell of food, and psychological states. When any one of these conditions is adversely affected, the stomach produces excess quantities of hydrochloric acid, which is called hyper-acidity, or less than normal quantity which is termed hypoacidity. Impulses received from the autonomic nervous system govern the acid production. The autonomic nervous system has two parts, called the sympathetic and the para-sympathetic, respectively. Their functions are the opposite of each other. The former stimu- the heart and lungs, releases more energy for use in lates the body, slows down the activity of digestion and assimilation, and thus prepares the body for taking quick action in an emergency. The result is fight or flight. The para-sympathetic on the other hand promotes conservation of energy and building up of tissues by stimulating digestion and assimilation of food, and its stor- age in the liver and tissues. When there is emotional disturbance due to anxiety, frustration, fear or disappointment, the balance between the sympathetic and para-sympathetic activities is dis- turbed. This is what happens in psychosomatic ailments.

Acidity is quite often psychosomatic in origin. Emotions of rage and fear may excite the sympathetic and adrenal systems, thus inhibiting the secretions of the stomach and bowels. This gives rise to hypoacidity. By the excitation of the para-sympa- thetic system due to jealousy, envy and frustrations, the gastro- intestinal functions are accelerated, resulting in hyperacidity.

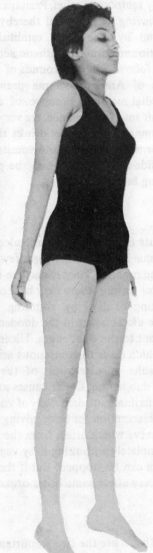

Fig. 60 : SHAVASANA : Lie down like a corpse. This asana relaxes the muscles and through them the mind, releasing tensions. Prescribed in hypertension.

REMEDY

When acidity has a psychosomatic origin, as is often the case, local treatment gives only temporary relief. Pranayama can bring a permanent cure by relieving tensions and thereby removing the cause of acidity and by once again establishing a balance between the sympathetic and para-sympathetic activities. Three rounds of Kapalabhati followed by ten rounds of bahya kumbhaka and twenty rounds of Anuloma-viloma pranayama with bandhas is an ideal remedial measure. Practice of asanas, vamana dhauti, and gulping air into the stomach are very useful additional techniques. In vamana dhauti one drinks three or four glasses of lukewarm water with little salt and vomits it out by putting the fingers deep inside the mouth. It may be practised in the morning before taking breakfast.

11. Gastric and peptic ulcers

Gastric ulcers may be acute or chronic. Chronic ulcers are painful. The pain may continue intermittently for a few weeks and vanish afterwards for some months. Then it may re-appear again. About two hours after eating there may be a burning pain. It can be relieved by taking alkali or by vomiting. There may also be heartburn. Peptic ulcers occur in the duodenum or the part of the stomach adjacent to the duodenum. Ulcers may have psychosomatic causes which leads to continuous acid production which ultimately results in ulceration of the inner lining of the stomach or the duodenum. Other causes are irregular food habits, mechanical irritants, or deficiency of vitamins. The stimulus for continuous secretion of acid, giving rise to ulcers comes from the vagus nerve which arises from the brain. If this nerve is blocked by completely sectioning it by vagotomy operation then ulcer formation can be stopped. But if the mental conflicts persist then they may affect some other organ.

REMEDY

Pranayama and vamana dhauti are the two important yoga techniques for cure of ulcers. Regulation of diet and habits is necessary. Alcohol is contra-indicated. Spices and chillies must be avoided. Milk and boiled vegetables may be taken.

12. Chronic dysentery

Dysentery is caused by contamination of food and drinks. Adulterated milk is a potent source of this disease. It is of two types: bacillary and amoebic. The former starts abruptly and is characterised by diarrohea, lower abdominal cramps, and watery stool often mixed with blood and mucus. There may be fever and dehydration. Amoebic dysentery is a chronic disease in which there is recurrence of diarrohea and abdominal cramps with semifluid stools containing blood-stained mucus.Frequently this may be associated with tenderness of the liver with enlargement. Quite often there is constipation, dyspepsia, fever, and general weakness. Drugs give temporary relief because the amoeba cannot be completely eradicated as protective cysts are formed as a reaction to drugs, and the micro-organism resists the drugs in this form.

REMEDY

Medical treatment must be taken when the attack is on. Pranayama with bandhas helps to make the system strong. Asanas involving forward and backward bending help the process. Instead of milk one should take yoghurt, curd, or buttermilk.

13. Piles

Piles is one of the most troublesome disorders which can better be prevented by doing pranayama than curing. Most persons suffering from piles are patients of chronic constipation. The waste matter not being evacuated properly and quickly accumulates for a long time in the rectum. It becomes dry and hard, and pressure is required to be applied for passing it out. Due to straining at stool, prolonged sitting or anal infection piles develop when the veins and the venous plexus at the anus get congested. There is rectal bleeding, protrusion, mucoid discharge from the rectum, and a feeling of discomfort. People with sedentary habits and doing no exercise are prone to get piles if they have constipation. Piles may be external or internal. External piles are more painful. In internal piles there is more bleeding.

REMEDY

When one becomes normal by medical or surgical treatment pranayama should be started. Care should be taken to remove constipation by regular exercise, walking, doing asanas, and regular eating habits. Kapalabhati, bahya kumbhaka, and twenty rounds of pranayama with bandhas should be practised once every day. One should eat enough vegetables, pectin containing fruits, and take enough fluids.

14. Hypertension

Hypertension or high blood pressure has become far more common in recent years than in the days of the generation of our parents. Normally the blood pressure of an average adult is 120 mm. Hg., when the left lower chamber of the heart contracts to force the blood through the arteries, and 80 mm. Hg. when this chamber expands to allow blood into it from the upper left chamber. The former is called systolic blood pressure and the latter diastolic blood pressure. With age the elasticity of the arteries is reduced and they become more rigid. So the heart is required to force the blood with greater force, and the blood pressure increases. In obese people the channels of the blood vessels get narrowed by deposition of fat inside them. This puts an additional pressure on the heart to pump the blood through the narrow channels. This is hypertension, which means that the heart is constantly exerting abnormally.

In all of us blood pressure does show a rise temporarily whenever there is physical activity, but it comes down to the normal level in a few minutes after the stress is over. In the case of a hypertensive it does not come down quickly.

Hypertension in many cases indicates an earlier stage of future cardiovascular disease. If hypertension is cured that means that an impending heart attack or myocardial infarction is averted or at least postponed considerably.

Hypertension is of two types: (i) primary or essential hypertension (ii) secondary hypertension. In the former type no specific cause for the rise in blood pressure can be ascertained. But it is found that there is usually an increase in the sympathetic activity. The majority of the cases of hypertension come under this category. Secondary hypertension is associated with disease of some other organ such as the kidneys, or tumors of the adrenal cortex or of the brain.

Hypertension causes undue fatigue due to little physical activity, giddiness, headache, dizziness and palpitation. There may be loss of breath with slight exertion.

REMEDY

In addition to drugs which bring down the blood pressure when it rises high, one may employ the yogic techniques with great advantage. They are: relaxation, bahya kumbhaka, and pranayama without inner kumbhaka. Relaxation should be done in Shavasana in a lying down position for twenty minutes in the morning and twenty minutes in the evening. This may be followed by ten rounds of bahya kumbhaka and twenty rounds of puraka and rechaka of ten and twenty seconds respectively. Mild exercise like walking may be taken to keep the body fit.

15. Varicose veins

Due to lack of exercise, obesity, and standing for a long time the venous circulation in the legs becomes slow and there is congestion of blood. The valves inside the veins become weak. There is much discomfort and pain in the legs.

REMEDY

In the sitting postures for pranayama the legs are folded and pressed. This helps to remove the congestion of blood in them. Pranayama of any variety promotes blood circulation. Practice of asanas having an inverted position, e.g. Shirshasana, Sarvangasana and Viparitakarani rests the valves in the veins and helps the flow of blood towards the heart due to gravity. Putting a strip of flannel or felt cloth tightly around the leg

below the knee gives support to the veins and helps to check
their distension. If one finds it difficult to practise the topsyturvy
postures then one may use a cushion below the feet so as to
keep the legs in an inclined position while sleeping, thus promoting circulation towards the heart.

16. Common cold, Rhinitis, and Sinusitis

All of us suffer from common cold some time or the other,
and although it is not a major disease it causes a lot of uneasiness and discomfort. It is often caused by infection of the
mucus membrane of the upper respiratory passage. There may
be running of the nose or choking of one or both nostrils, and
irritation of the mucus membrane due to inflammation. In
rhinitis there is watery nasal discharge, hypersensitivity of the
mucus membrane, and nasal congestion. Often there is eosinophilia and itching of the nasal mucosa.

The sinuses are air spaces which communicate with the
cavity of the nose. During a severe cold, the inflammation
often spreads from the mucus lining of the nose to the lining
of the sinuses, causing headache and pain between the eyes.
Sinus infection causes pain, swelling, headache, fever, and
nasal congestion. If not treated in time, it may become chronic.
Many people suffer again and again from attacks of cold and
sinusitis, due to hypersensitivity of the inner lining to dust
particles, paints, perfumes, and pollen grains from the flowers
of various species. This is called allergy. In the absence of the
allergen there is no trouble. But contact with it may often
produce symptoms just in a few minutes.

REMEDY

Antihistaminic drugs give quick relief by blocking the
action of histamine which is a toxic product released in the
reaction of a tissue to an allergen. But a better way is to
remove the hypersensitivity of the mucus membrane, which
can be achieved by a regular practice of Kapalabhati, pranayama and neti. Three rounds of Kapalabhati followed by
twenty rounds of Suryabhedana pranayama would be an ideal

remedy for the above troubles. Sutraneti should be practised every day for two to three weeks, and then twice a week.

17. Chronic Bronchitis

The wind pipe or trachea divides into two branches going to the two lungs. These are called the bronchi. Chronic bronchitis is a disease of the bronchi caused by inflammation of the mucus lining and adjoining tissue. Dampness, dust pollution, and smoking aggravate it. The disease is more pronounced in winter. Prolonged affection may cause loss of elasticity of the bronchi. The lungs may also become rigid and cannot expand and contract fully. There is cough and sticky sputum. The elastic tissue becomes fibrous, causing difficulty in respiration. Older people are affected more.

REMEDY

Kapalabhati and pranayama offer the best preventive measures. In the case of an attack medical treatment should be taken, and when one becomes normal pranayama should be practised every day. Neti and dhauti should be practised occasionally. Asanas of the keep fit yoga routine should be done.

18. Asthma

There are two types of asthma. Cardiac asthma is caused by acute ventricular failure. Pranayama and other yoga techniques are of no avail for it. The other type is bronchial asthma. This is more common and amenable to yogic treatment. Bronchial asthma is a disorder of hypersensitivity of the bronchi and their branches. It has a strong hereditary character. Allergy to dust, pollen, and other forms of allergens is often associated with the attacks of asthma. Histamine released into the blood gives rise to spasms of the respiratory tract. Eosinophilia is also noticed. In many cases psychological factors are involved. Due to narrowing of the respiratory passage there is great difficulty in breathing out. Wheezing and gasping for breath is very common. Constipation, choking in the nose, eczema, and neurodermatitis are often observed to accompany asthma.

REMEDY

While the attack is on no yoga techniques can be practised. Immediate relief can be had by medical treatment. When one becomes normal again, Kapalabhati, bahya kumbhaka, pranayama with bandhas, and asanas may be practised. Ujjayi, Anuloma-viloma or Suryabhedana pranayama should be practised. Pranayama makes the respiratory system strong, helps to remove congestion and accumulated secretions from the respiratory tract, and cleans the respiratory passage. Vamana dhauti should be practised every day when an attack is expected. The technique of a hot foot bath as prescribed in nature cure also helps a great deal.

19. Nervousness and Instability of Mind

It is necessary to have a capacity to take quick and firm decisions for success in life. Many persons lack this capacity, and are nervous and fussy. They change their decisions repeatedly, often putting themselves into awkward situations. This is actually a psychological problem which can be solved to a certain degree by psychological counselling. A regular practice of pranayama is observed to help a great deal in training the mind and making it firm and stable.

20. Sciatica

The sciatic nerve is situated at the back side of the thigh. Dividing itself into two, it goes down the leg. It is formed by the union of the upper three sacral nerves and the lumbodorsal trunk. Sciatica means pain associated with this nerve. It may be caused by pressure on the nerve, inflammation, or due to spondylitis. Sometimes the trouble arises from minor causes like sitting on the angular edge of a chair or any hard surface. Or while lifting a heavy load the nerve might be strained. Sometimes stumbling causes sciatica by straining the nerve. Pranayama offers a good remedy by exercising the trunk and the lower limbs in the sitting posture. Among the asanas one may practise Bhadrasana, Gomukhasana, and Paschimottanasana.

21. Insomnia

Sleep is a phenomenon common to all of us. But none of us can tell what it is and how it comes. We sleep in parts, moving the body a number of times during sleep, there being various stages coming and doing, such as, dreaming, half waking state, deep sleep, and so on. We have waves of sleep rather than a stream of sleep. The waves are interrupted by tensions in the body and mind. The depth of sleep is more important for giving rest to the body. When the disturbing factors get an upper hand, one cannot get enough rest during sleep, and there is still a lingering feeling of fatigue and heaviness when one gets up. This is what happens in insomnia.

Sleeplessness is on the increase now a days because of the complexities of daily life and the tensions created by them. Drugs do induce deep sleep, but they have side effects. Moreover, one's dependence on them goes on increasing as one goes on taking drugs, and the size of the dose is also required to be increased as the habit grows.

REMEDY

In a recent study of the treatment of insomnia made by the present writer ("Treatment of Insomnia through Yoga and Nature Cure Techniques", *Yoga Awareness Journal*, Vol. IV. no. 3., August 1980, pp. 30-35) it was found that the extent of sleep during the night was very significantly increased in case of twenty patients with treatment for one month which included a daily practice of the following: (i) Yoga postures for 20 minutes, (ii) guided relaxation for 15 minutes, (iii) deep breathing through alternate nostrils for 10 minutes, (iv) meditation of Hamsajapa for 10 minutes, (v) spinal bath of cold water for 20 minutes, and (vi) hot foot bath in the end before going to sleep, for five minutes.

In the above study the relative effect of each of the techniques for increasing sleep was not measured. But in the follow up studies after the patients gave up the practices taught to them during the experiment except asanas, pranayama and guided relaxation, which they could do without external help, it was found that the gain in sleep was maintained at a study level. So it may be recommended that one should practise asanas of the keep fit yoga routine for 20 minutes, then pranayama with or without kumbhaka for ten minutes in the evening and then before going to bed relaxation for 15 minutes in the bed. This helps to get good sleep.

22. Spondylitis

The cause of this disease is unknown. It is frequently observed to be familial. It is observed to be much more prevalent in men than in women. Spondylitis begins with backache radiating down the thighs. Morning stiffness with sharp catching pain in the back not relieved by rest is a marked feature of the disease. As it progresses pain and stiffness moves upward along the spine, restricting the movement of the affected joints. There is inflammation of the intervertebral ligaments. The chest cannot be expanded fully. Later on the vertebral bodies may fuse together. Advanced cases are called bamboo spine, where even slight bending on any side becomes impossible due to stiffening of joints.

REMEDY

Asanas involving backward bending, use of moist heat for relaxation and massage form the main line of treatment of spondylitis. Taking salt free diet, fasting, and liquid diet may also be used with advantage. Pranayama may be started when the joints become free again. If done in the initial stages of the disease, pranayama can stop further deterioration and advance of the disease.

23. Rheumatoid arthritis

Unlike spondylitis this is a disease which prefers women to men. It affects the smaller joints first and later on the bigger joints. Initially there are vague aches and pains. Then gradually swelling appears in the joints, accompanied by pain. There may be morning stiffness and fatigue, and tenderness of joints Joints of the hands, feet, and knees are more commonly affected. Movement of the affected joint becomes limited and painful.

Emotional disturbances, repressed disagreeable emotions, and faulty diet are some of the main causes of rheumatoid arthritis.

REMEDY

Like many other disorders this can also be very effectively prevented by doing pranayama. But when the disorder sets in it may not be possible to practise pranayama easily. Asanas which would give progressive resistance exercise to the joints and limbs provide the best remedy. Such asanas are : Gomukhasana, Bhadrasana, Uttanamandukasana, Halasana and Bhujangasana. Heat and cold treatment, fasting, and massage would also be useful.

24. Gout

This is a disease which prefers meat eating people much more to vegetarians. Uric acid, which is an end product of protein metabolism, accumulates in the joints as monosodium urate when one eats lots of animal proteins. It causes inflammation and pain. With constantly high uric acid level of the blood the kidneys may be adversely affected. Gout involves the joints of hands, feet, and synovial joints, where crystals of sodium urate accumulate in the synovial cavity. This causes pain.

REMEDY

Pranayama acts better as a preventive measure. Asanas giving corrective exercise to the affected parts and joints should be practised. Movements of the joints while holding a topsy-turvy pose gives good relief. Elimination of excess protein from the diet is essential. Massage and application of moist heat as in steam bath is very useful.

25. Displacement of the uterus

Sometimes during child birth there is injury to the pelvic floor, especially affecting the transverse cervical and uterosacral ligaments. This often results in retroversion of the uterus and prolapse. This may be painful and may affect further child bearing. Retroversion can be prevented and checked by doing pranayama with bandhas. Practice of asanas like Bhadrasana, Gomukhasana, Uttanamandukasana, Yogamudra, Paschimatana, and Matsyasana is very useful for bringing the uterus to the correct position again. Ashvini mudra and Mula bandha have a special significance for this purpose.

26. Irregularities of menstruation

Menstruation is uterine bleeding which occurs at intervals of 24 to 32 days in the normal woman during the reproductive years. Ovulation and the resulting production of estrogen and progesterone hormones results in bleeding, when pregnancy does not occur. The beginning of menstrual periods, which generally occurs between 11 and 14 years of age, is called menarche, while the menopause or cessation of menstruation occurs between 45 and 55 years of age.

Irregularities of menstruation may indicate disease or deficiency states or emotional disturbance or hormonal imbalance. Excessive bleeding during the normal time is called hypermenorrohea. Prolonged bleeding is called menorrhagia. Painful menstruation or dysmenorrhea is characterised by cramps in the lower abdomen and discomfort. Metrorrhagia means irregular flow at times other than the normal menstrual period. In olygomenorrhea there is scanty discharge.

All these irregularities of menstruation can very well be prevented and checked by pranayama and *asanas*. But it is always good to have medical check up done first to ascertain the cause of irregularity. If the trouble is due to infection or hormonal imbalance then medical treatment must be taken.

27. Sexual weakness

The reproductive system has two functions: to perpetuate the species, and to give sex pleasure or sexual enjoyment. Sexual weakness may hamper both these functions. Infertility or impotence is an extreme example of sexual weakness. Pranayama and asanas can be of great help in overcoming various forms of sexual weakness in a majority of cases Kapalabhati followed by bahya kumbhaka (ten rounds) and Anuloma-viloma pranayama with bandhas should be practised once every day. Among the asanas Shirshasana, Sarvangasana, and Paschimatana are important for this purpose. Ashvini-mudra and Nauli should be practised every day. All these techniques are very useful for increasing the strength of the muscles associated with the sex function, in both male and female.

28. Maladjustment of personality

Many of us are physically well off but mentally ill adjusted. Our life is largely a matter of relationship, and how we respond in this relationship to various things, persons and beliefs is an expression of our personality. Happiness in life depends on these responses. To be a well adjusted person means to have contentment and satisfaction, restraint on our desires and consideration for others, and peace and stability of mind. Maladjustment of personality expresses itself in the form of anxiety, irritability, harmful habits like smoking, alcoholism, and criminality.

If all of man's desires could be fulfilled then there would be no conflict in the world and no tensions. But such a thing has never so far been possible, and we always find that there is a gap between our desires and their fulfilment. All our efforts in life are directed in the ultimate analysis to fill the gap between the 'desired' and the 'actual'. If the gap is too wide then life becomes a struggle. Happiness depends on two factors. One is the gap itself, and the other is how we react to it, accept it, and adjust ourselves with it. Science tries to bridge this gap between what we desire and what we actually have by its inventions, discoveries and technological advances. But it

176 YOGIC PRANAYAMA

does not teach us how to bring about a happy adjustment
between our desires and what the world has to offer us. This
task of adjusting our behaviour with the surroundings has
traditionally been handled by religion and philosophy. But
with the progress of science in the recent past many beliefs
held very dearly by religion and philosophy have been
questioned. The result is that the influence which these two
disciplines used to have on our minds is greatly reduced. This
has given rise to an imbalance between our inner and outer
worlds. Science enriches the outer world, and it has done this
most wonderfully. But enrichment of the inner world is lagging
behind because the two disciplines which took care of it in the
past have failed and nothing has taken charge in their place.
That is why in this scientific age we see so much maladjustment of personality.

Our inner nature is dominated by some universally present
innate tendencies and attitudes. Interest in one's own existence
and that of the species, likes and dislikes, and fulfilment of
biological urges, are some of these tendencies which are ingra-
ined in us. All our behaviour in daily life issues from these
tendencies. They are of course necessary for life. The inner-
outer balance depends on keeping these tendencies within
certain limits. If they go out of hand they definitely disturb
the balance. For instance, self-interest is very essential for life,
but when it grows excessively due to lack of restraint it creates
no end of trouble for the individual and for others.

Unrestrained animal nature expresses itself in the form of
anxiety, greed, envy, hate, exploitation, and other vices. Bad
habits like drinking and smoking are also an expression of lack
of restraint of the animal tendencies.

Pranayama, as we have explained earlier, makes an ideal
programme for training of the mind and promoting restraint
of the animal nature. The present writer had an opportunity to
be associated with an experiment in which hardened criminals
serving long terms in a Central Jail were given training in
asanas and pranayama for a period of three months. The
results were very encouraging. A remarkable change was
observed in the attitudes of the participants. Clashes between
the convicts were reduced, and pessimism, emotional outbursts
and irritability were conspicuously reduced. An important

observation of the jail authorities was that a feeling of self confidence, co-operative attitude and poise was evident in the behaviour of those who completed the course.

It is an experience of the present writer that in scores of cases regular practice of pranayama resulted into giving up almost completely the habits of smoking and drinking excessively.

These examples suggest that pranayama can bring about remarkable changes in one's personality by establishing an inner-outer balance. On the basis of our present knowledge we may not be able to explain how all the beneficial changes are brought about. But one thing seems to be certain from the experience so far, namely, that pranayama as a key to good physical and mental health deserves the attention of every one who cares for health and happiness in life.

□ □

Appendix

A Keep Fit Yoga Routine

Apart from pranayama there are many other techniques of yoga such as asanas, mudras, and kriyas which have a great significance for maintenance of good health. They have much utility in preventing and curing disorders. A minimum course called 'keep fit yoga routine' which the present writer has taught to thousands of yoga enthusiasts with very good results is given below. In all it requires about 60 minutes including relaxation, pranayama and meditation. If one cannot give this much time at a stretch then the routine may be divided into two parts, doing pranayama and meditation in the morning and other techniques in the evening. Following is the order of practice.

1. Bhadrasana with bandhas...1 minute.
2. Uttanamandukasana with bandhas...1 minute.
3. Gomukhasana—three stages......3 minutes.
4. Sarala Matsyendrasana (both sides) . .2 minutes.
5. Ushtrasana with Simha mudra......$\frac{1}{2}$ minute.
6. Yoga mudra ....1 minute.
7. Matsyasana......1 minute.
8. Viparitakarani... .2 minutes.
9. Sarvangasana... .1 minute.
10. Halasana...2 minutes.
11. Bhujangasana...1 minute.
12. Shalabhasana... .1 minute
13. Dhanurasana... .1 minute.
14. Chakrasana... .$\frac{1}{2}$ minute.
15. Shirshasana... .2 minutes.
16. Relaxation in Shavasana... . .10 minutes.
17. Bahya kumbhaka (10 rounds)...10 minutes.

18. Pranayama......10 minutes.
19. Meditation (Hamsajapa)... .10 minutes.

If the routine is divided into two parts, the asanas and
relaxation may be given thirty minutes in the evening, and
pranayama and meditation, thirty minutes in the morning. If on
some occasions the time is short then all the techniques may be
done in the same order, giving less time to each one.

□ □ □